A to Z of Venous Thromboembolism

A to Z of Venous Thromboembolism: A Thesaurus

V.K. Kapoor
Professor, Surgical Gastroenterology
Sanjay Ghandi Post-Graduate Institute
of Medical Sciences
Lucknow, India

S.K. Das
Consulting Vascular and Endovascular Surgeon
Hillingdon Hospital NHS Foundation Trust
and London North West University Health
Care NHS Trust
London, UK

Forewords by
Prof V.V. Kakkar (Deceased)
OBE, FRCS, FRCSE, Hon DSc
London, UK

Rt Hon Lord A.K. Kakkar
Director, Thrombosis Research Institute
London, UK

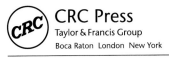

CRC Press
Taylor & Francis Group
Boca Raton London New York

CRC Press is an imprint of the
Taylor & Francis Group, an **informa** business

Second edition published 2021
by CRC Press
6000 Broken Sound Parkway NW, Suite 300, Boca Raton, FL 33487-2742

and by CRC Press
2 Park Square, Milton Park, Abingdon, Oxon, OX14 4RN

© 2021 Taylor & Francis Group, LLC
First edition published by Medeka Health Private Limited 2012
CRC Press is an imprint of Taylor & Francis Group, LLC

ISBN: 9780367753009 (hbk)
ISBN: 9780367220334 (pbk)
ISBN: 9780429270413 (ebk)

Typeset in Minion Pro
by KnowledgeWorks Global Ltd.

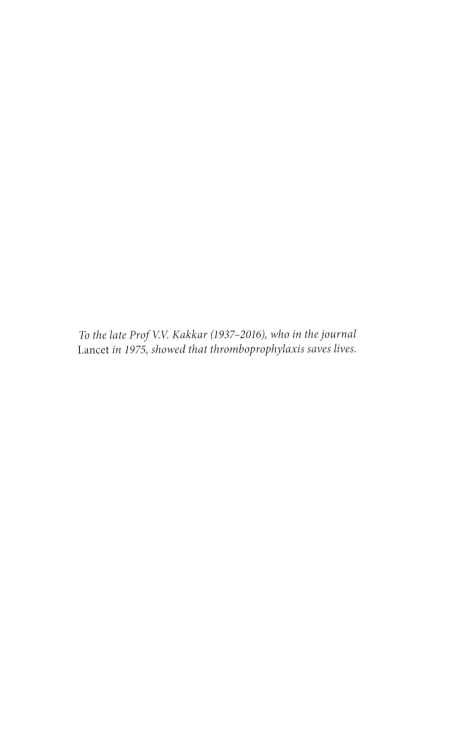

To the late Prof V.V. Kakkar (1937–2016), who in the journal Lancet *in 1975, showed that thromboprophylaxis saves lives.*

CONTENTS

Suggested Readings

Brands of Thromboprophylaxis Agents

Index

FOREWORD

Despite over 50 years of intense research effort with substantial advances in our understanding of the pathophysiology, diagnosis, natural history and methods for the prevention and treatment of venous thromboembolism (VTE), it still remains a major cause of morbidity and mortality in health systems throughout the world. The continuing focus on the need to apply routine risk assessment for VTE amongst hospitalized patients and the provision of robust guidelines for its prevention remains essential.

The substantial global research effort which continues to inform advances in the development of anticoagulant therapy essential for the management of VTE and innovation in novel techniques to further improve outcomes in patients with extensive deep vein thrombosis is essential. In their quick reference monograph (*A to Z of Venous Thromboembolism*), Vinay Kapoor and Saroj Das provide an invaluable aid for clinicians and healthcare professionals to establish the foundations of understanding which is essential in helping them to improve clinical outcomes for their patients.

Rt Hon Lord A.K. Kakkar
Professor of Surgery
University College, London
Director, Thrombosis Research Institute
London, UK

FOREWORD TO THE FIRST EDITION

Venous thromboembolism (VTE) is a major cause of death and disability in our society. Though the research for an effective method of prophylaxis against VTE has been ongoing for nearly 90 years, a method that is effective in the total elimination of this condition is yet to be developed. This uninspiring state of affairs has been due, firstly, to a lack of essential knowledge of a trigger mechanism which initiates blood clotting and, secondly, the nonavailability of a simple method of prophylaxis which can be used to protect high-risk patients from fatal pulmonary embolism.

The last 40 years have seen a resurgence of dedicated attempts to develop such a method, and this has been possible due to an understanding of the chemical structure, mode of action and advances in separating various fractions of heparin. This has led to the development of low-molecular-weight-heparin (LMWH) prophylaxis.

During the last 20 years, LMWHs have served us well in clinical practice. They are easy to administer and, in most cases, do not require laboratory monitoring and have thus proved to be highly effective and safe in the prophylaxis and treatment of VTE, and their use is likely to increase over the coming years.

This quick reference monograph by Prof V.K. Kapoor will provide useful information relating to VTE for busy physicians and thus stimulate the widespread use of VTE prophylaxis in clinical practice in India, which is most urgently needed.

Emeritus Professor V.V. Kakkar
3 November 2010
OBE, FRCS, FRCSE, Hon DSc
Director, Thrombosis Research Institute
Emmanuel Kaye Building, Manresa Road
Chelsea, London, UK

PREFACE

It is well known that safe surgery saves lives; safer surgery will, therefore, save more lives. Safe surgery includes not only a skilled operative procedure but also adequate preoperative preparation and close postoperative care. Some complications of surgery are unavoidable, but many can be prevented. One of the easily preventable complications of surgery is deep venous thrombosis (DVT) and its dreaded sequela – pulmonary embolism (PE).

The development of our knowledge about venous thromboembolism (VTE) can be described in three phases: past, present and future. Thanks to the pioneering work carried out by the late Professor V.V. Kakkar and others through landmark clinical trials and research, we now have a comprehensive understanding about the epidemiology and natural history of venous thromboembolism (VTE) in different populations, different ethnic groups and people from different geographic backgrounds. Since Jay McLeans's observation (1916) about the role of heparin in the treatment of thrombosis, we have learnt about controlling the disease and preventing the morbidity and mortality due to VTE. The unravelling of the myth behind clotting cascades unfolded and simplified our knowledge about clotting activation and thrombolysis. We also learnt about vulnerable people at high risk of developing VTE. These are the 'known knowns' that were revealed by opening the Pandora's box.

During the last two decades, we explored the 'known unknowns': the risk assessment for VTE, developing imaging modalities, pharmaco-mechanical and ultrasonic energy for thrombus debulking and use of stenting in venous compression syndromes; identifying the high-risk groups that may need intensive and extended treatment; and new drug development. There were trials and tribulations that led to excitement, hope and despair. Many of the new drugs like hirudin, ximelagatran, idraparinux and heparinoids were abandoned from further research development and were excluded from clinical use due to significant side effects. Millions of dollars were wasted in their development, but such is the price we have to pay for new drug development. More promising drugs appeared on the scene, and it was expected that these compounds will change the way we manage our patients with VTE; it will be simpler, cheaper and will have minimal side effects. The direct oral anticoagulants (DOACs) are such compounds that showed lots of promise. Antidotes were developed to counteract their bleeding side effects. However, they have not yet shown their full potential, and warfarin continues to dominate the scene in the treatment of VTE. Therefore, it appears that there is a large vacuum in our research that has not yet addressed our quest for an ideal anticoagulant.

That brings us to the future: the exploration of the 'unknown unknowns'. There are many tasks that we need to undertake: (1) finding an ideal anticoagulant; (2) challenging the natural history of the disease in the light of societal changes, people's behaviour and attitude towards life; (3) changing the pattern of chronic diseases; and (4) managing cancer- and chemotherapy-associated VTE.

The medical students of the future generations will need to be taught on a holistic platform to enhance their learning need and to engage in high-class research in the making of a good doctor. This will include: (1) molecular biology and genetic profiling, (2) molecular modelling, (3) exchanging and sharing research and networking using digital technology, (4) medical professionalism, (5) minimally invasive surgery and (6) developing personalized treatment and target-specific treatment. The objective of this exercise will be to deliver a seamless, enjoyable and risk-free journey for our patients in the future.

Thromboprophylaxis has been proven and documented to be the number-one measure to ensure the safety of hospitalized patients. It is up to the practicing physicians and surgeons to adopt this measure with an aim to improve the safety of our patients – the prime objective of our profession and practice.

We have made a small attempt to pen down a few facts and some figures about VTE with an intent to make a practicing physician (and surgeon) aware of the entity and existence of VTE and the efficacy and safety of thromboprophylaxis. We will consider our effort to have been worthwhile if even one life is saved by the use of thromboprophylaxis after reading this book.

V.K. Kapoor
Lucknow, India
vkkapoor.india@gmail.com
http//vkkapoor-india.weebly.com

S.K. Das
London, UK
saroj.das@imperial.ac.uk

"All doctors treat diseases,
good doctors diagnose disease early,
the best doctors prevent diseases."

ACKNOWLEDGEMENTS

I am grateful to Drs Gaurav Agrawal, S.K. Agrawal, Afzal Azeem, A.K. Baronia, Anu Behari, Deepak Dubey, Priti Elhence, Rakesh Kapoor, Rajesh Kashyap, R.K. Singh, Aneesh Srivastava and P.K. Srivastava for contributing to various CME programmes on VTE organized by me and sponsored by Astra Zeneca, Elder, GSK, Pfizer, Piramal and Sanofi Aventis.

I am also grateful to Dr Ammar Raza (Astra Zeneca), Dr Amit Bhargava (Elder Pharmaceuticals), Dr Vrishali R. Desai (GSK), Dr Shalini Menon (Pfizer), Dr Srikumar Chattopadhyay (Piramal) and Dr Manish Hathial (Sanofi Aventis) for their valuable input and comments on the manuscript of the 1st edition.

Acknowledgements are due to Ms Varsha Yadav, VTE research assistant, and Mr K.K. Srivastava for typing the manuscript.

V.K. Kapoor

SPECIAL ACKNOWLEDGEMENT

We are specially grateful to Prof Ajay Khanna of the Department of Surgery at the Institute of Medical Sciences (IMS) in the Banaras Hindu University (BHU), Varanasi, India, (Editor. Venous Disorders. Springer: 2018) for reviewing the final manuscript and making valuable additions and suggestions.

We are grateful to Himani Dwivedi, Shivangi Pramanik and Mouli Sharma at Taylor & Francis of India, Kyle Meyer at Taylor & Francis USA and Nancy Rebecca at Cenveo for their help in the production of this monograph.

V.K. Kapoor
S.K. Das

ACKNOWLEDGEMENT FOR IMAGES
Dr Brijesh Singh, SGPGIMS, Lucknow (Figs. I1, V1, V3, V5)

Dr Saurabh Galodha, AIIMS, New Delhi (Figs. I2, U1)

Dr Shivani Rao, Indira Gandhi Medical College, Shimla (Figs. C5, P5)

ABOUT THE AUTHORS

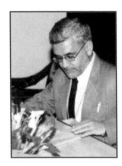

Dr V.K. Kapoor is a professor of surgical gastroenterology at the Sanjay Gandhi Post-Graduate Institute of Medical Sciences (SGPGIMS), Lucknow, India. Prof Kapoor has been a visiting professor to the Oregon Health and Science University (OHSU), Portland, Oregon, USA; the King's College Hospital (KCH), London, UK; and the International Medical University (IMU), Kuala Lumpur, Malaysia, and a visiting consultant surgeon to the Zayed Military Hospital (ZMH), Abu Dhabi, UAE. He has been an examiner for the Intercollegiate MRCS at the Royal Colleges of Surgeons of England, Edinburgh and Glasgow, UK, the University Kebangsan Malaysia (UKM), Kuala Lumpur, Malaysia; Anna Medical College, Mauritius; BP Koirala Institute of Health Sciences (BPKIHS), Dharan, Nepal; and Health Authority of Abu Dhabi (HAAD), Abu Dhabi, UAE. Dr Kapoor has been awarded the Fulbright Fellowship, Commonwealth Fellowship, Scholarship of the International College of Surgeons, Clinical Oncology Fellowship of the UICC and Fellowship of the German Academic Exchange Service (DAAD). He has also been awarded the ICMR International Fellowship, DBT Overseas Associateship and Dr B.C. Roy Award (Medical Council of India). Prof Kapoor has been an invited speaker at international conferences and at institutions in Australia, Austria, Bangladesh, Bhutan, Chile, China, Czech Republic, Dominican Republic, Egypt, France, Germany, Hong Kong, Japan, Malaysia, Mauritius, Nepal, Oman, Pakistan, Peru, Poland, Russia, Singapore, South Korea, Sri Lanka, Switzerland, Thailand, Turkey, UAE, UK and the United States. In addition to having published books on clinical surgery, safe cholecystectomy, gall bladder cancer, bile duct injury and acute pancreatitis, Prof Kapoor has also authored a quiz book on Mahatma Gandhi.

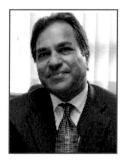

Dr S.K. Das is a consulting vascular and endovascular surgeon at the Hillingdon Hospital NHS Foundation Trust and London North West University Health Care NHS Trust, London, UK. He is also an honorary professor at the Brunel Institute of Bioengineering, London, and honorary senior lecturer and director of clinical studies at the Imperial College of Science, Technology and Medicine, London, UK. He completed his MBBS from the Utkal University, India, and MS from the All India Institute of Medical Sciences (AIIMS), New Delhi, India. He is a member of the National Board of Examinations (NBE). He then obtained an FRCS (Glasgow and England) and M Phil (National Heart & Lungs Institute, University of London). He also has a diploma in laparoscopic surgery from the University of Strasbourg, France. He has been a visiting consultant surgeon at the Waikato Hospital, Hamilton, New Zealand; the Westmead Hospital, Sydney, Australia; and at the Arizona Heart Institute, Phoenix, Arizona, USA. Dr Das is the Regional Specialty Professional Advisor (RSPA), College Assessor for the Advisory Appointment Committee and Regional Director for London at the Royal College of Surgeons of England (RCSE). He is an examiner for MRCS at the RCSE and for FRCS at the Joint Committee for Intercollegiate Examinations. Dr Das was the honorary secretary, Vascular Medicine, and currently he is the president of Vascular Lipid Metabolic Medicine (LVMM) at the Royal Society of Medicine (RSM). Dr Das has been a course director at the Asia Pacific Vascular Intervention Course (APVIC), New Delhi, India, and on the faculty of the Charing Cross International Vascular Symposium, London, UK; Moroccan Society of Vascular Surgery, FRCS course; London Deanery; and Medicines Sans Frontiers (MSF). He is the chairman of the medical student selection panel at the Imperial Medical School, London, and a member of the selection panel for surgical trainees and foundation trainees. Dr Das is a fellow of the Asia Pacific Vascular Society, Edward Dietrich Vascular Surgical Society, European Society of Vascular and Endovascular Surgery, International Society of Endovascular Surgery, International Society of Thrombosis and Haemostasis, Society of Academic and Research Surgeons and Vascular Society of Great Britain and Ireland.

LIST OF ABBREVIATIONS

ACCP	American College of Chest Physicians
aPTT	Activated partial thromboplastin time
BID	Twice daily
CT	Computed tomography
CUS	Compression ultrasonography
CVC	Central venous catheter
DOAC	Direct oral anticoagulants
DUS	Doppler ultrasonography
DVT	Deep venous thrombosis
FUT	Fibrinogen uptake test
GCS	Graduated compression stockings
HFS	Hip fracture surgery
HIT	Heparin-induced thrombocytopenia
INR	International normalized ratio
IPC	Intermittent pneumatic compression
IVC	Inferior vena cava
LDUH	Low-dose unfractionated heparin
LMWH	Low-molecular-weight heparin
MI	Myocardial infarction
NOAC	Novel (non–vitamin K antagonist) oral anticoagulant
OD	Once daily
PAH	Pulmonary arterial hypertension
PE	Pulmonary embolism
PPS	Post-phlebitic syndrome
PTS	Post-thrombotic syndrome
SC	Subcutaneous
SCI	Spinal cord injury
THA	Total hip arthroplasty
THR	Total hip replacement
TID	Thrice daily
TKA	Total knee arthroplasty
TKR	Total knee replacement
UFH	Unfractionated heparin
VFP	Venous foot pump
VKA	Vitamin K antagonist
VTE	Venous thromboembolism – deep venous thrombosis (DVT) + pulmonary embolism (PE)

KEY POINTS ABOUT
VENOUS THROMBOEMBOLISM

- Venous thromboembolism (VTE) is common in hospitalized patients, even in Asia and India.
- VTE is usually underestimated.
- VTE is usually silent and difficult to diagnose and treat.
- VTE can be dangerous – even fatal.
- Fatal pulmonary embolism (PE) can be the very first manifestation of (asymptomatic, silent) deep vein thrombosis (DVT).
- VTE is easy to prevent – PE is the most common preventable cause of hospital deaths.
- VTE prophylaxis is highly effective, largely safe and extremely cost-beneficial.
- VTE prophylaxis reduces the risk of VTE but does not completely abolish it.
- VTE prophylaxis is the number-one strategy for the safety of hospitalized patients and extended prophylaxis in the community in some high-risk conditions.
- VTE prophylaxis, unfortunately, is highly underutilized and needs to be used more often in indicated patients.
- There is a need to be aware of and alert about VTE in all patients.
- All patients should be evaluated for their risk for VTE and given thrombo-prophylaxis accordingly.
- Each hospital should have its own protocol and policy for preventing VTE.

FREQUENTLY ASKED QUESTIONS ABOUT VENOUS THROMBOEMBOLISM

Does venous thromboembolism (VTE) occur in India?

The belief that VTE does not occur in Indian patients is a myth; there are enough data to show that VTE occurs in Indian patients also and is probably as common as in the West.

Is VTE harmful?

VTE is dangerous and can be fatal also. Long-term **sequelae** of VTE can adversely affect the quality of life (QoL) of patients.

Why not screen for VTE instead of prophylaxis?

Routine screening of all patients with ultrasonography (US) for VTE is logistically difficult and is not cost-effective. Detection of VTE by screening would involve treatment with a high dose of anticoagulation, with the morbidity and mortality associated with it, whereas VTE prophylaxis with a small dose of anticoagulation is associated with fewer complications.

Why not detect VTE at an early stage and treat it?

In the majority of cases, VTE is silent (asymptomatic) and therefore difficult to diagnose. Moreover, early diagnosis of VTE needs venography – an invasive investigation.

Why not treat VTE when it occurs?

Deep vein thrombosis (DVT) itself may be asymptomatic (silent), and VTE may present for the first time as a pulmonary embolism (PE). Treatment of VTE involves full dose therapeutic anticoagulation (cf. thromboprophylaxis) with potential for serious bleeding complications.

Can VTE be prevented?

There is enough strong evidence that thromboprophylaxis reduces the incidence of DVT, PE and fatal PE.

Which patients are at risk for VTE?

Elderly, obese, critically ill, hospitalized, those with cancer and those undergoing major (>45 minutes) surgery and those with **thrombophilia**.

How can VTE be prevented?

The quantum of the risk of VTE can be estimated. VTE prophylaxis includes mechanical and pharmacological measures. Pharmacological measures of prophylaxis have been documented to be the most effective; mechanical measures add to their benefit.

Can VTE still occur in patients receiving VTE prophylaxis?

Yes, because VTE prophylaxis reduces the risk of VTE but does not completely abolish it.

Which heparin should be used for prophylaxis of VTE?

Either unfractionated heparin (UFH) or low-molecular-weight heparin (LMWH) can be used, but LMWH is preferred over UFH.

How? How much?

Subcutaneous

Prophylactic doses are less than the therapeutic doses.

Are dose schedules different for the LMWHs?

UFH needs to be administered 2–3 times a day; LMWHs need only once-a-day dose.

Are there any patients in whom pharmacological thromboprophylaxis is contraindicated?

Patients with active bleeding, patients with a lesion which can potentially bleed e.g. peptic ulcer, patients with coagulopathy. In brain and spine surgery, mechanical prophylaxis is preferred over pharmacological agents.

When to start? How long?

Preoperative (2–12 hours) or postoperative (12 hours).

The duration depends on the risk of VTE; it is usually 7–14 days, but some patients may require extended (4–5 weeks) prophylaxis.

Is VTE prophylaxis safe?

VTE prophylaxis is associated with either no or little increase in major bleeding. Special precautions are required, however, if spinal/epidural anaesthesia is used.

What are the risks of VTE prophylaxis?

Thromboprophylaxis causes little or no increase in the risk of clinically important bleeding. Appropriate use of thromboprophylaxis has a favourable benefit/risk ratio.

Does VTE prophylaxis need monitoring?

Prophylactic doses of anticoagulants do not require coagulation profile monitoring. Platelet counts, however, need to be checked.

Is VTE prophylaxis cost-effective?

Thromboprophylaxis has been proven to be the number-one strategy to improve the safety of hospitalized patients in both the United States and Europe. It decreases the overall costs of management.

SOME MYTHS/MISCONCEPTIONS ABOUT VENOUS THROMBOEMBOLISM

(WHICH, OBVIOUSLY, ARE NOT TRUE)

- Venous thromboembolism (VTE) occurs in the West only and does not occur in India. (It does occur in India too.)
- VTE occurs in hospitalized patients only and does not occur in outpatients. (VTE can and does occur in patients who do not require hospitalization – more so in those with thrombophilia.)
- If the patient is ambulant, she or he does not require thromboprophylaxis. (Immobilization is one of several, and not the only, risk factors for VTE. Even ambulant patients may be at risk of VTE and need thromboprophylaxis if other risk factors are present.)
- VTE occurs in critically ill patients admitted to the intensive care unit (ICU) and does not occur in patients admitted to the general wards. (VTE is certainly more common in patients admitted to the ICU but does occur in non-ICU patients also.)
- VTE occurs in surgical patients only and does not occur in medical patients. (VTE occurs in medical patients also, especially those admitted to the ICU.)
- VTE occurs in bed-ridden patients only and does not occur in ambulatory patients. (VTE can occur in ambulatory patients also.)
- The risk of VTE is only as long as the patient is admitted in the hospital, and there is no risk after the patient is discharged. (The risk of VTE may continue even after discharge from the hospital.)
- Only elderly patients are at risk for VTE – young patients don't have a risk of VTE. (VTE is frequent in young patients also.)
- Mechanical methods of thromboprophylaxis can be used in place of pharmacological prophylaxis. (They do not replace, but rather complement, each other.)
- Pharmacological thromboprophylaxis is associated with a higher risk of bleeding. (There is no or very little increased risk of clinically significant bleeding with the use of pharmacological prophylaxis.)

- Unfractionated heparin (UFH) is as good as low-molecular-weight heparin (LMWH). (Yes, they are equally effective but LMWH is better than UFH in high-risk patients. Furthermore, LMWH has a better biological response and side effect profile than UFH. LMWH requires once a day dose vs. 2–3 doses a day for UFH.)
- Only those cancer patients who require chemotherapy are at a risk for VTE. (All cancer patients, with or without chemotherapy, are at increased risk of VTE.)

GLOBAL VENOUS THROMBOEMBOLISM GUIDELINES

AAFP (AMERICAN ACADEMY OF FAMILY PHYSICIANS)

https://www.aafp.org/afp/2017/0301/p295.html

AAOS (AMERICAN ASSOCIATION OF ORTHOPEDIC SURGERY)

https://www.aaos.org/quality/quality-programs/tumor-infection-and-military-medicine-programs/venous-thromboembolic-disease-in-elective-tka-and-tha-prevention/

ACCP (AMERICAN COLLEGE OF CHEST PHYSICIANS)

Evidence-based clinical practice guidelines.

Bates SM, Jaeschke R, Stevens SM, Goodacre S, Wells PS, Stevenson MD, Kearon C, Schunemann HJ, Crowther M, Pauker SG, Makdissi R, Guyatt GH. Diagnosis of DVT: Antithrombotic therapy and prevention of thrombosis, 9th ed: American College of Chest Physicians Evidence-Based Clinical Practice Guidelines. *Chest.* 2012;141(Suppl 2):e351S–418S. doi: 10.1378/chest.11-2299. PMID:22315267

Kahn SR, Lim W, Dunn AS, Cushman M, Dentali F, Akl EA, Cook DJ, Balekian AA, Klein RC, Le H, Schulman S, Murad MH. Prevention of VTE in non-surgical patients: Antithrombotic therapy and prevention of thrombosis, 9th ed: American College of Chest Physicians Evidence-Based Clinical Practice Guidelines. *Chest.* 2012;141(Suppl 2):e195S–226S. doi: 10.1378/chest.11-2296. PMID:22315261

Kearon C, Akl EA, Comerota AJ, Prandoni P, Bounameaux H, Goldhaber SZ, Nelson ME, Wells PS, Gould MK, Dentali F, Crowther M, Kahn SR. Antithrombotic therapy for VTE disease: Antithrombotic therapy and prevention of thrombosis, 9th ed: American College of Chest Physicians Evidence-Based Clinical Practice Guidelines. *Chest.* 2012;141(Suppl 2):e419S–96S. doi: 10.1378/chest.11-2301. Erratum in: *Chest.* 2012 Dec;142(6):1698–1704. PMID:22315268

Gould MK, Garcia DA, Wren SM, Karanicolas PJ, Arcelus JI, Heit JA, Samama CM. Prevention of VTE in nonorthopedic surgical patients: Antithrombotic therapy and prevention of thrombosis, 9th ed: American College of Chest Physicians Evidence-Based Clinical Practice Guidelines. *Chest.* 2012;141(Suppl 2):e227S–e277S. doi: 10.1378/chest.11-2297. PMID: 22315263

API (ASSOCIATION OF PHYSICIANS OF INDIA)

http://apiindia.org/wp-content/uploads/pdf/medicine_update_2010/cardiology_31.pdf

ASCO (AMERICAN SOCIETY OF CLINICAL ONCOLOGY)

https://www.asco.org/research-guidelines/quality-guidelines/guidelines/supportive-care-and-treatment-related-issues%20#/9911

Key NS, Bohlke K, Falanga A. Venous Thromboembolism Prophylaxis and Treatment in Patients With Cancer: ASCO Clinical Practice Guideline Update Summary. *J Oncol Pract.* 2019;15(12):661–64. doi: 10.1200/JOP.19.00368. Epub 2019 Sep 24. No abstract available. PMID:31550210

Key NS, Khorana AA, Kuderer NM, Bohlke K, Lee AYY, Arcelus JI, Wong SL, Balaban EP, Flowers CR, Francis CW, Gates LE, Kakkar AK, Levine MN, Liebman HA, Tempero MA, Lyman GH, Falanga A. Venous thromboembolism prophylaxis and treatment in patients with cancer: ASCO Clinical Practice Guideline Update. *J Clin Oncol.* 2020;38(5):496–520. doi: 10.1200/JCO.19.01461. Epub 2019 Aug 5. PMID:31381464

ASH (AMERICAN SOCIETY OF HEMATOLOGY)

Lim W, Le Gal G, Bates SM, Righini M, Haramati LB, Lang E, Kline JA, Chasteen S, Snyder M, Patel P, Bhatt M, Patel P, Braun C, Begum H, Wiercioch W, Schünemann HJ, Mustafa RA. American Society of Hematology 2018 guidelines for management of venous thromboembolism: diagnosis of venous thromboembolism. *Blood Adv.* 2018;2(22):3226–56. doi: 10.1182/bloodadvances.2018024828. PMID:30482764

ASRA (AMERICAN SOCIETY OF REGIONAL ANESTHESIA)

Horlocker TT, Vandermeulen E, Kopp SL, Gogarten W, Leffert LR, Benzon HT. Regional anesthesia in the patient receiving antithrombotic or thrombolytic therapy: American Society of Regional Anesthesia and Pain Medicine Evidence-Based Guidelines (Fourth Edition). *RegAnesth Pain Med.* 2018;43(3):263–309. doi: 10.1097/AAP.0000000000000763

AUSTRALIAN COMMISSION ON SAFETY AND QUALITY IN HEALTH CARE

https://www.safetyandquality.gov.au/our-work/clinical-care-standards/venous-thromboembolism-prevention-clinical-care-standard

EAU (EUROPEAN ASSOCIATION OF UROLOGY)

https://uroweb.org/guideline/thromboprophylaxis/

ESMO (EUROPEAN SOCIETY OF MEDICAL ONCOLOGY)

https://www.esmo.org/guidelines/supportive-and-palliative-care/venous-thromboembolism-vte-in-cancer-patients

EUROPEAN SOCIETY OF CARDIOLOGY

https://www.revespcardiol.org/en-vol-68-num-1-sumario-S1885585714X00137

ITAC (INTERNATIONAL INITIATIVE ON THROMBOSIS AND CANCER)

https://www.itaccme.com/en

IUA (INTERNATIONAL UNION OF ANGIOLOGY)

Cardiovascular Disease Educational and Research Trust; Cyprus Cardiovascular Disease Educational and Research Trust; European Venous Forum; International Surgical Thrombosis Forum; International Union of Angiology; Union Internationale de Phlébologie. Prevention and treatment of venous thromboembolism. International Consensus Statement (guidelines according to scientific evidence). *Int Angiol.* 2006; 25(2):101–61. PMID: 16763532.

NCCN (NATIONAL COMPREHENSIVE CANCER NETWORK)

https://www.nccn.org/

NICE (NATIONAL INSTITUTE FOR HEALTH AND CARE EXCELLENCE)

https://www.nice.org.uk/guidance/ng89

RCOG (ROYAL COLLEGE OF OBSTETRICIANS AND GYNAECOLOGISTS)

https://www.rcog.org.uk/globalassets/documents/guidelines/gtg-37a.pdf

SAGES (SOCIETY OF AMERICAN GASTROINTESTINAL AND ENDOSCOPIC SURGEONS)

VTE prophylaxis for laparoscopic surgery guidelines.

https://www.sages.org/publications/guidelines/guidelines-for-deep-venous-thrombosis-prophylaxis-during-laparoscopic-surgery/

SIGN (SCOTTISH INTERCOLLEGIATE GUIDELINES NETWORK)

Prophylaxis of venous thromboembolism, 2002.
https://www.sign.ac.uk/media/1060/sign122.pdf

AAFP (AMERICAN ACADEMY OF FAMILY PHYSICIANS)
https://www.aafp.org/afp/2017/0301/p295.html

AAOS (AMERICAN ASSOCIATION OF ORTHOPEDIC SURGERY)
Clinical Practice Guideline on Preventing Venous Thromboembolic Disease in Patients Undergoing Elective Hip and Knee Arthroplasty
   https://www.aaos.org/quality/quality-programs/tumor-infection-and-military-medicine-programs/venous-thromboembolic-disease-in-elective-tka-and-tha-prevention/

ABDOMINAL SURGERY
DVT can occur in as many as 10%–25% and PE in 2% of patients undergoing abdominal surgery without thromboprophylaxis.

ABG (ARTERIAL BLOOD GASES)
Hypoxia (low PaO_2), detected on arterial blood gases (ABG), is present in most patients with PE, but there are several other causes for hypoxia i.e. poor specificity; also, normal PaO_2 does not rule out PE i.e. poor sensitivity.

ABPI (ANKLE–BRACHIAL PRESSURE INDEX)
The ankle–brachial pressure index (ABPI) is recorded by measuring the systolic pressure in the ankle arteries e.g. dorsalis pedis and posterior tibial artery and in the brachial artery. Normal value is 0.9–1.1. Low (<0.9) ABPI indicates arterial disease e.g. atherosclerosis.

ACC (ACUTE CORONARY CARE)
Most patients admitted to the acute coronary care (ACC) unit will require thromboprophylaxis.

ACCP (AMERICAN COLLEGE OF CHEST PHYSICIANS)
American College of Chest Physicians Guidelines

Bates SM, Jaeschke R, Stevens SM, Goodacre S, Wells PS, Stevenson MD, Kearon C, Schunemann HJ, Crowther M, Pauker SG, Makdissi R, Guyatt GH. Diagnosis of DVT: Antithrombotic therapy and prevention of thrombosis, 9th ed: American College of Chest Physicians evidence-based clinical practice guidelines. *Chest.* 2012;141(2 Suppl):e351S–e418S. doi: 10.1378/chest.11-2299. PMID:22315267

A

Gould MK, Garcia DA, Wren SM, Karanicolas PJ, Arcelus JI, Heit JA, Samama CM. Prevention of VTE in nonorthopedic surgical patients: Antithrombotic therapy and prevention of thrombosis, 9th ed: American College of Chest Physicians evidence-based clinical practice guidelines. *Chest.* 2012;141(2 Suppl):e227S–e277S. doi: 10.1378/chest.11-2297. PMID: 22315263

Kahn SR, Lim W, Dunn AS, Cushman M, Dentali F, Akl EA, Cook DJ, Balekian AA, Klein RC, Le H, Schulman S, Murad MH. Prevention of VTE in nonsurgical patients: Antithrombotic therapy and prevention of thrombosis, 9th ed: American College of Chest Physicians evidence-based clinical practice guidelines. *Chest.* 2012;141(2 Suppl):e195S–e226S. doi: 10.1378/chest.11-2296. PMID: 22315261

Kearon C, Akl EA, Comerota AJ, Prandoni P, Bounameaux H, Goldhaber SZ, Nelson ME, Wells PS, Gould MK, Dentali F, Crowther M, Kahn SR. Antithrombotic therapy for VTE disease: Antithrombotic therapy and prevention of thrombosis, 9th ed: American College of Chest Physicians evidence-based clinical practice guidelines. *Chest.* 2012;141(2 Suppl):e419S–e496S. doi: 10.1378/chest.11-2301. Erratum in: *Chest.* 2012 Dec;142(6):1698–1704. PMID:22315268

ACENOCOUMAROL
Oral vitamin K antagonist (**VKA**), a **coumarin** derivative.

ACQUIRED
Acquired risk factors for VTE include surgery, **trauma**, immobilization, medical illnesses, etc.

ACS (ACUTE CORONARY SYNDROME)
Patients with acute coronary syndrome (ACS) need anticoagulation **treatment** (NOT just **prophylaxis**).

ACTIVATED PROTEIN C RESISTANCE
This is a hypercoagulable state characterized by the lack of a response to activated protein C (APC), which normally helps prevent blood from clotting excessively.

ACTIVITY
Activity of the LMWHs is expressed as their **anti-Xa** activity.

ADMISSION
In the United States, thromboprophylaxis is usually started after (NOT before) surgery to enable the patient to be admitted on the day of the surgery.

ADVERSE EVENTS
Risk of adverse events e.g. **bleeding**, heparin-induced thrombocytopenia (**HIT**), heparin-induced thrombocytopenia and thrombosis syndrome (**HITTS**) and osteoporosis are less with LMWHs than with UFH.

AGE

The risk of VTE increases with increasing age. In the **Caprini** score, age 41–60 years has 1 point, 61–74 years 2 points and ≥75 years has 3 points. Age >60 years has been found to have odds ratio (OR) of 2–6 for VTE. Incidence of VTE in those aged 70–79 years is 300–500 per 100,000 cf. about 30 per 100,000 for those aged 25–35 years.

Young (<40 years) patients are usually thought not to be at risk of VTE and are not even considered for prophylaxis. They may, however, have additional risk factors e.g. **cancer**, **major surgery**, **thrombophilia**, etc., which may put them at risk for VTE.

AIDA (ASSESSMENT OF INCIDENCE OF DVT IN ASIA)

It was thought that VTE is a 'Western' disease and does not occur or is uncommon in **Asian** ethnic populations. A prospective epidemiological study in 19 centres across Asia (China, Indonesia, Malaysia, Philippines, South Korea, Taiwan and Thailand), however, showed a 41% incidence of DVT (proximal DVT in 10%) in 837 patients undergoing elective total hip replacement (**THR**), total knee replacement (**TKR**) or hip fracture surgery (**HFS**) without pharmacological thromboprophylaxis.

Piovella F, Wang CJ, Lu H, Lee K, Lee LH, Lee WC, Turpie AG, Gallus AS, Planès A, Passera R, Rouillon A; AIDA investigators. Deep-vein thrombosis rates after major orthopedic surgery in Asia. An epidemiological study based on postoperative screening with centrally adjudicated bilateral venography. *J Thromb Haemost*. 2005;3(12):2664–70. doi: 10.1111/j.1538-7836.2005.01621.x.PMID: 16359505

AIMS OF TREATMENT

The aims of treatment of DVT are to:

1. Halt the extension of the thrombus in the vein
2. Prevent or reduce pulmonary embolism from the thrombus
3. Prevent or reduce post-thrombotic syndrome (**PTS**), **recurrent** DVT and pulmonary arterial hypertension (**PAH**)

AIR TRAVEL

Long-distance (>6 hours) air travel may predispose to VTE, especially in the presence of other risk factors. Precautions include nonrestrictive clothing, adequate hydration, avoiding excess alcohol, exercise i.e. leg exercise, calf massage and ankle mobilization, walking before and after travel and during the stop-overs. Patients with a risk factor may use high-pressure (20–25 mm Hg) graduated compression stockings (**GCS**) or even receive prophylactic LMWH.

A

AMBULATION

Ambulation activates the calf muscle pump.

1. Patients waiting for elective surgery should be instructed to remain ambulant, and early ambulation should be encouraged after the operation to reduce the risk of VTE.
2. Early ambulation, along with graduated compression stockings (**GCS**), is recommended in patients with established DVT.
3. Early aggressive frequent ambulation alone is enough for young (<40 years) patients with no risk factors.

AMERICAN ACADEMY OF FAMILY PHYSICIANS (AAFP)

See **AAFP**.

AMERICAN ASSOCIATION OF ORTHOPEDIC SURGERY (AAOS)

See **AAOS**.

AMERICAN SOCIETY OF CLINICAL ONCOLOGY (ASCO)

See **ASCO**.

AMERICAN SOCIETY OF HEMATOLOGY (ASH)

See **ASH**.

AMERICAN SOCIETY OF REGIONAL ANESTHESIA (ASRA)

See **ASRA**.

ANAESTHESIA

1. Vasodilatation during anaesthesia results in venous stasis in the lower limbs, thus increasing the risk of VTE.
2. Duration of anaesthesia >2 hours has odds ratio (OR) of 4–5 for VTE.

ANGIOGRAPHY

Pulmonary angiography is the gold standard for the diagnosis of PE – conventional invasive angiography is rarely used now; CT pulmonary angiography (**CTPA**) and MR pulmonary angiography (**MRPA**) are preferred. Dilated pulmonary arteries with sudden tapering on angiography support the diagnosis of PE.

AngioJet™

AngioJet (Boston) is a DVT **thrombectomy** catheter to treat large (>6 mm diameter) veins.

ANTIDOTE
Protamine is an antidote for UFH, and it partly reverses the action of LMWHs as well; however, there is no antidote for **fondaparinux**. Antidotes are now available for some of the direct oral anticoagulants (**DOACs**). An antidote for **dabigatran** is available in India, but it is very expensive. No antidote is available for the other **DOACs**.

ANTINEOPLASTIC EFFECT
Heparin has some antineoplastic effect because of the inhibition of micro-thrombi, tumour cell adhesion and angiogenesis. LMWHs, when used for the treatment of VTE, have shown to improve the prognosis in cancer patients in clinical trials.

ANTIPLATELET DRUGS
Antiplatelet drugs e.g. **aspirin**, **clopidogrel**, **dipyridamole**, ticlopidine are more useful for arterial thrombosis e.g. coronary artery disease (CAD), **stroke**, transient ischemic attacks (TIA), etc., but do not have a role in VTE prophylaxis. However, in a collaborative meta-analysis of randomized trials of antiplatelets, **aspirin** alone was found to be effective in reducing the incidence of PE.

ANTITHROMBIN (ANTI-IIa) AGENTS
Dabigatran and **melagatran** are new antithrombin (**anti-IIa**) agents; they are also called direct thrombin inhibitors (**DTIs**).

Ximelagatran has been withdrawn from clinical use due to hepatic toxicity.

ANTITHROMBIN 3
Deficiency of antithrombin 3 (as also of **protein C and S**) are risk factors for VTE.

ANTITHROMBOTIC DRUGS
Antithrombotic drugs include both anticoagulants (i.e. **heparins**, **anti-Xa agents** and **warfarin**) and **antiplatelet drugs**.

ANTI-IIa AGENTS
See **Antithrombin agents**.

ANTI-Xa AGENTS
Fondaparinux and **idraparinux** are selective anti-Xa agents. Some new oral anti-Xa drugs e.g. **apixaban, edoxaban** and **rivaroxaban** are now being used in the treatment of VTE.

ANTI-Xa ASSAY

Anti-Xa assay is the best method to monitor therapeutic anticoagulation but is not practical and is not generally used in clinical practice.

ANTI-Xa TO ANTI-IIa RATIO

Factor Xa plays a central role in the coagulation process – both intrinsic and extrinsic pathways. Factor Xa activates the conversion of factor II (**prothrombin**) to factor IIa (**thrombin**). Thrombin (IIa) then converts **fibrinogen** to **fibrin**. Fibrin, along with the red blood cells (RBCs), forms the clot (thrombus).

A higher anti-Xa to anti-IIa ratio leads to greater antithrombotic activity without an increased risk of bleeding. **Bemiparin** has the highest (8:1) anti-Xa to anti-IIa ratio, followed by **parnaparin** (4.0:1), **enoxaparin** (3.8:1), **nadroparin** (3.0:1), **dalteparin** (2.7:1) and **tinzaparin** (1.9:1); UFH (1:1) has the least anti-Xa to anti-IIa ratio. The WHO recommends the anti-Xa to anti-IIa ratio to be at least 2.5.

API (ASSOCIATION OF PHYSICIANS OF INDIA)

An Indian perspective on VTE published by the Association of Physicians of India (API)

http://apiindia.org/wp-content/uploads/pdf/medicine_update_2010/cardiology_31.pdf

APIXABAN

Apixaban is a direct oral anticoagulant (**DOAC**) – it is a selective factor Xa inhibitor. It is approved for:

1. Prevention of VTE in adults undergoing total hip replacement (**THR**) or total knee replacement (**TKR**) – started 12–24 hours AFTER surgery – 2.5 mg PO thrice daily for 30–35 days (THR) or for 10–14 days (TKR)
2. Treatment of VTE 10 mg PO BD or TID × 7 days followed by 5 mg PO BD or TID
3. Prevention of recurrent VTE 2.5 mg PO TID after 6 months of treatment of VTE
4. Prevention of **stroke** in patients with atrial fibrillation.

APOLLO TRIAL

In 1,309 patients undergoing major abdominal surgery, **fondaparinux**, when combined with intermittent pneumatic compression (**IPC**), reduced the incidence of VTE from 5.3% to 1.7% when compared with IPC alone (459 patients in each arm); any bleeding (15, 2.4% vs. 4, 0.6%) and major bleeding (10, 1.6% vs. 1, 0.2%) was, however, more common with the use of fondaparinux.

Turpie AG, Bauer KA, Caprini JA, Comp PC, Gent M, Muntz JE; Apollo Investigators. Fondaparinux combined with intermittent pneumatic compression vs. intermittent pneumatic compression alone for prevention of venous thromboembolism after abdominal surgery: A randomized, double-blind comparison. *J Thromb Haemost*. 2007;5(9):1854–61. doi: 10.1111/j.1538-7836.2007.02657.x.PMID: 17723125

aPTT (ACTIVATED PARTIAL THROMBOPLASTIN TIME)

Activated partial thromboplastin time (aPTT) is used to monitor therapeutic heparinization with UFH – it is maintained at 1.5–2.5 times the control value. There is no normal aPTT, as the value varies from lab to lab, depending upon the reagents used. aPTT is not as prolonged with LMWHs as with UFH due to their low **anti-IIa** activity. aPTT monitoring is not required when heparins (UFH or LMWH) are used in prophylactic doses and when LMWH and the direct oral anticoagulants (**DOAC**s) are being used for the treatment of VTE.

ARDS (ADULT RESPIRATORY DISTRESS SYNDROME)

The clinical picture and even radiological appearance (on **chest X-ray** or CT) of adult respiratory distress syndrome (ARDS) may mimic those of PE. ARDS, however, is usually bilateral, whereas PE is more commonly unilateral.

ARGATROBAN

Argatroban is a synthetic inhibitor of **thrombin** (factor IIa) – a direct thrombin inhibitor (**DTI**). It can be used for prophylaxis and treatment of VTE in patients with heparin-induced thrombocytopenia (**HIT**). Because of its hepatic metabolism, it may be used in patients with renal dysfunction.

ARRIVE

In a multicentre retrospective registry involving 549 patients with a confirmed diagnosis of VTE – deep vein thrombosis (DVT) confirmed by Doppler ultrasonography and pulmonary embolism (PE) confirmed by computed tomography (CT), pulmonary angiography and/or **V/Q scan** at three tertiary care hospitals in India from 2006 to 2010 – acute DVT without PE, acute DVT with PE and PE alone were reported in 64% (352/549), 23% (124/549), and 13% (73/549) of patients, respectively. Surgery, including orthopaedic surgery (28%); **trauma** (16%); and **immobilization** >3 days (14%) were the most common risk factors for VTE.

Kamerkar DR, John MJ, Desai SC, Dsilva LC, Joglekar SJ. ARRIVE: A retrospective registry of Indian patients with venous thromboembolism. *Indian J Crit Care Med*. 2016;20(3):150–58. doi:10.4103/0972-5229.178178

ARTEMIS

No symptomatic VTE occurred when **fondaparinux** was used in acutely ill **medical patients** (cf. fatal PE in 1.2% patients in the placebo group). VTE rates were 5.6% in the fondaparinux group vs. 10.5% in the placebo group.

Cohen AT, Davidson BL, Gallus AS, Lassen MR, Prins MH, Tomkowski W, Turpie AG, Egberts JF, Lensing AW; ARTEMIS Investigators. Efficacy and safety of fondaparinux for the prevention of venous thromboembolism in older acute medical patients: Randomized placebo controlled trial. *BMJ.* 2006;332(7537):325–29. doi: 10.1136/bmj.38733.466748.7C. Epub 2006 Jan 26.PMID: 16439370

ARTHROPLASTY

Total hip and knee arthroplasty (replacement) (**THR** and **TKR**) patients are at very high risk for VTE. Fatal PE can occur in 5% of patients undergoing arthroplasty without VTE prophylaxis.

ASCO (AMERICAN SOCIETY OF CLINICAL ONCOLOGY)

https://www.asco.org/research-guidelines/quality-guidelines/guidelines/supportive-care-and-treatment-related-issues%20#/9911

Key NS, Bohlke K, Falanga A. Venous thromboembolism prophylaxis and treatment in patients with cancer: ASCO clinical practice guideline update summary. *J Oncol Pract.* 2019;15(12):661–64. doi: 10.1200/JOP.19.00368. Epub 2019 Sep 24. No abstract available. PMID:31550210

Key NS, Khorana AA, Kuderer NM, Bohlke K, Lee AYY, Arcelus JI, Wong SL, Balaban EP, Flowers CR, Francis CW, Gates LE, Kakkar AK, Levine MN, Liebman HA, Tempero MA, Lyman GH, Falanga A. Venous thromboembolism prophylaxis and treatment in patients with cancer: ASCO clinical practice guideline update. *J Clin Oncol.* 2020;38(5):496–520. doi: 10.1200/JCO.19.01461. Epub 2019 Aug 5. PMID:31381464

ASH (AMERICAN SOCIETY OF HEMATOLOGY)

Lim W, Le Gal G, Bates SM, Righini M, Haramati LB, Lang E, Kline JA, Chasteen S, Snyder M, Patel P, Bhatt M, Patel P, Braun C, Begum H, Wiercioch W, Schünemann HJ, Mustafa RA. American Society of Hematology 2018 guidelines for management of venous thromboembolism: Diagnosis of venous thromboembolism. *Blood Adv.* 2018;2(22):3226–56. doi: 10.1182/bloodadvances.2018024828. PMID:30482764

ASIAN

Many studies have reported lower rates of DVT in Asian populations as compared to Western populations. A prospective epidemiological study in 19 centres across Asia (China, Indonesia, Malaysia, Philippines, South Korea, Taiwan and Thailand), however, showed a 41% incidence of DVT (proximal DVT in 10%) in 837 patients undergoing elective total hip replacement (**THR**), total knee replacement (**TKR**) or hip fracture surgery (**HFS**) without pharmacological thromboprophylaxis.

Piovella F, Wang CJ, Lu H, Lee K, Lee LH, Lee WC, Turpie AG, Gallus AS, Planès A, Passera R, Rouillon A; AIDA investigators. Deep-vein thrombosis rates after major orthopedic surgery in Asia. An epidemiological study based on postoperative screening with centrally adjudicated bilateral venography. *J Thromb Haemost.* 2005;3(12):2664–70. doi: 10.1111/j.1538-7836.2005.01621.x. PMID: 16359505

ASPIRIN (ACETYL SALICYLIC ACID)

Acetyl salicylic acid (aspirin), a nonsteroidal anti-inflammatory drug (NSAID), has **antiplatelet** properties and is useful for arterial (NOT venous) thrombosis. It reduces the risk of myocardial infarction (**MI**) and **stroke**. Aspirin alone cannot be used for VTE prophylaxis. It is NOT recommended as a primary modality of VTE prophylaxis in any of the **guidelines**.

ASRA (AMERICAN SOCIETY OF REGIONAL ANESTHESIA)

ASRA guidelines (2002) for the use of **neuraxial** anaesthesia in patients receiving pharmacological thromboprophylaxis.

https://www.asra.com/advisory-guidelines/article/9/regional-anesthesia-in-the-patient-receiving-antithrombotic-or-thrombolytic-ther

Horlocker TT, Vandermeulen E, Kopp SL, Gogarten W, Leffert LR, Benzon HT. Regional anesthesia in the patient receiving antithrombotic or thrombolytic therapy: American Society of Regional Anesthesia and Pain Medicine evidence-based guidelines (fourth edition). *Reg Anesth Pain Med.* 2018;43(3):263–309. doi: 10.1097/AAP.0000000000000763

ASYMPTOMATIC DVT

Asymptomatic (**silent**) DVT (detected by screening **Doppler** US) is about 5–10 times more common than symptomatic DVT. Even extensive DVT may be asymptomatic. The risk of PE is greater in patients with asymptomatic DVT than in patients with symptomatic DVT. This is possibly because symptomatic DVT is more likely to be detected and treated with anticoagulation, thus decreasing the risk of PE, whereas patients with asymptomatic DVT are more likely to remain undiagnosed and not to receive any anticoagulation, thus increasing their risk of developing PE.

ATTRACT

The Acute Venous Thrombosis: Thrombus Removal with Adjunctive Catheter-Directed Thrombolysis (ATTRACT) trial provided evidence to support catheter-directed **thrombolysis** (**CDT**) for the management of ilio-femoral DVT.

Vedantham S, Goldhaber SZ, Julian JA, Kahn SR, Jaff MR, Cohen DJ, Magnuson E, Razavi MK, Comerota AJ, Gornik HL, Murphy TP, Lewis L, Duncan JR, Nieters P, Derfler MC, Filion M, Gu CS, Kee S, Schneider J, Saad N, Blinder

M, Moll S, Sacks D, Lin J, Rundback J, Garcia M, Razdan R, Vander Woude E, Marques V, Kearon C; ATTRACT trial investigators. Pharmacomechanical catheter-directed thrombolysis for deep-vein thrombosis. *N Engl J Med.* 2017;377(23):2240–52. doi: 10.1056/NEJMoa1615066. PMID: 29211671; PMCID: PMC5763501.

AT-RISK

One alternative option to prophylaxis is to screen at-risk patients and diagnose (and treat) DVT, but it is not as cost-effective as compared to thromboprophylaxis.

AUTOPSY

Autopsy studies show that a large number of DVT and PE remains unsuspected, undetected and untreated. PE was found in 32% of 1,234 hospitalized surgical patients who died and underwent autopsy. PE was the cause of death in 29% of these cases; it contributed to death in 27% and was incidental in 44%.

PE was found at autopsy in 59 of 404 (15%) patients. It caused or contributed to death in 22 of 59 (37%) and was incidental in 37 of 59 (63%). Among the patients at autopsy who died from PE, the diagnosis was unsuspected in 14 of 20. In these patients, death from PE occurred within 2.5 hours in 13 of 14.

11% prevalence of PE at autopsy.

See also **PGIMER.**

Lindblad B, Eriksson A, Bergqvist D. Autopsy-verified pulmonary embolism in a surgical department: Analysis of the period from 1951 to 1988. *Br J Surg.* 1991;78(7):849–52. doi: 10.1002/bjs.1800780725.PMID: 1873716

Stein PD, Henry JW. Prevalence of acute pulmonary embolism among patients in a general hospital and at autopsy. *Chest.* 1995;108(4):978–81. doi: 10.1378/chest.108.4.978.PMID: 7555172

Sweet III PH, Armstrong T, Chen J, Masliah E, Witucki P. Fatal pulmonary embolism update: 10 years of autopsy experience at an academic medical center. *JRSM Short Rep.* 2013;4(9):2042533313489824

A-V IMPULSE SYSTEM

A foot compression device (**FCD**).

AWARENESS

Lack of awareness about the incidence and the dangers of VTE and about the **safety** and efficacy of thromboprophylaxis are the main reasons for **underutilization** of VTE prophylaxis in clinical practice.

BALANCE
While using thromboprophylaxis, a balance has to be struck between the efficacy (i.e. prevention of VTE) on the one hand and the **safety** (i.e. risk of **bleeding**) on the other.

BALLOON
Endovascular balloon (Fig. B1) dilatation and stent placement can be used for opening the veins narrowed by thrombosis.

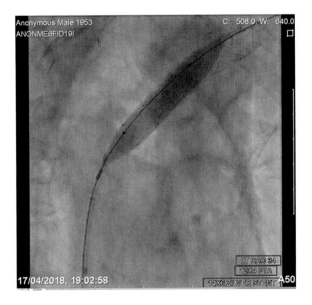

Fig. B1 Endovascular balloon dilatation of a narrowed vein. A stent will be placed after the dilatation.

BARIATRIC SURGERY
Obese patients undergoing bariatric surgery should receive thromboprophylaxis based on their total body weight (TBW).

BED REST

Bed rest >4 days has odds ratio (OR) of 4–5 for VTE.

BEGINNING

DVT usually begins in a calf vein and then extends to a **proximal** (i.e. ilio-femoral) vein; proximal DVT alone, without calf DVT, is rare. Proximal DVT is more likely to cause PE than distal DVT.

BEMIPARIN

Bemiparin is a second-generation LMWH. It has a low (3,600 Da) mean molecular weight, long (5.3 hours) half-life and high (8:1) **anti-Xa/anti-IIa** ratio. It is given as a once-daily (OD) dose started 2 hours before or 6 hours after surgery.

The dose for prophylaxis of VTE is 2,500–3,500 IU SC OD started 2 hours before or 6 hours after surgery.

The dose for the treatment of VTE is 115 IU per kg (5,000–7,500 IU) SC OD.

BIOMARKERS

Several biomarkers e.g. **D-dimer**, factor VIII, fibrin monomer, inflammatory cytokines, leukocyte count, microparticles, p-Selectin, etc., can predict DVT.

BIOPSY

A recent internal organ e.g. liver, kidney, biopsy is a contraindication for the use of the heparins.

BLEEDING

Fear of bleeding is the most common reason for not using thromboprophylaxis. Use of heparins (UFH or LMWH) in prophylactic dose is, however, associated with very low risk of significant bleeding. Minor bleeds e.g. injection site bruising, wound **hematoma** and drain site bleed are not uncommon (occurring in about 2%–3% of cases). Meta-analysis of randomized controlled trials has shown no or little increase in the rates of clinically important bleeding after prophylaxis with LMWH.

In the **PRIME** study, no patient in the **enoxaparin** group ($n = 477$) and only two (0.4%) in the UFH group ($n = 482$) had severe bleeding. Major bleeding also occurred less frequently in patients who received enoxaparin than in those who received UFH (2, 0.4% vs. 7, 1.5%).

Bleeding necessitates discontinuation of the pharmacological prophylaxis. Bleeding while on anticoagulation may be treated with fresh blood, vitamin K and **fresh frozen plasma** (FFP), and **protamine** may be given to neutralize overdose. In surgical patients, a surgical cause of bleeding should also be kept in mind.

Lechler E, Schramm W, Flosbach CW. The venous thrombotic risk in nonsurgical patients: epidemiological data and efficacy/safety profile of a low-molecular-weight heparin (enoxaparin). *The Prime Study Group Haemostasis*. 1996; 26(Suppl 2):49–56. doi: 10.1159/000217272. PMID: 8707167

B

BLEEDING INDEX
[No. of units of blood or packed red blood cells (RBCs) transfused] + [pre-bleeding Hb – post-bleeding Hb in Gm/dL]

BMI
Higher (>30) body mass index (BMI) is a risk factor for VTE.

B-MODE US (ULTRASONOGRAPHY)
B-mode US combined with **Doppler**, called a **duplex** scan, is the most important tool for making a diagnosis of DVT. A normal vein appears dark (echolucent), while a thrombosed vein is light (echogenic) on B-mode US.

BNP
Higher levels of brain natriuretic peptide (BNP) in patients with PE predict a higher risk of mortality.

BODY WEIGHT
The dosage of LMWH is based on the body weight of the patient. Caution should be exercised while using the heparins and **fondaparinux** in patients with body weight <50 kg.

BREAST CANCER
The 5-year incidence of VTE in patients with breast cancer who are on **tamoxifen** and chemotherapy is 4.2% vs. 0.9% in those on tamoxifen alone and 0.2% in those who are not on any of these.

The risk of VTE is less with the use of aromatase inhibitors e.g. anastrozole, letrozole than with tamoxifen.

BRIDGE THERAPY
Bridge therapy is an overlapping therapy between injectable and oral anticoagulants.

LMWH (e.g. **enoxaparin** 1 mg/kg SC BD or **dalteparin** 100 IU/Kg SC BD) is started and **warfarin** (5 mg oral) or **acenocoumarol** (4 mg oral) is started on day 3–5 and PT/INR is monitored. The **overlap** of heparin (UFH or LMWH) and warfarin lasts usually for 2–3 days.

B

For long-term prophylaxis, warfarin (with monitoring of **INR**, which should be maintained at 2–3) is given on an outpatient basis for 12 weeks. Warfarin may be replaced with direct oral anticoagulants (**DOAC**s).

Similarly, LMWHs can be used to bridge the interruption of **oral anticoagulants** in patients in whom anticoagulants have to be discontinued for some time for performing some invasive procedure. This is because it takes 2–3 days for the effect of **warfarin** to wane, whereas only 12–24 hours are required for the elimination of the effect of LMWH.

BURDEN

It is estimated that VTE causes a financial burden of about $1.5 billion per year in the United States.

BURNS

Patients with burns, who have additional risk factors for VTE, should receive VTE thromboprophylaxis.

C

C (protein)
Protein C is a zymogen; its activated form plays a role in regulating anticoagulation. Deficiency of protein C (as also protein **S**) is a risk factor for recurrent venous thromboembolism (VTE).

CALF CIRCUMFERENCE
Calf circumference should be monitored in both legs 10 cm below the tibial tuberosity to detect subtle unilateral leg oedema, an early sign of DVT.

CALF THROMBI
Distal (calf) thrombi detected on routine **screening Doppler** are usually clinically **asymptomatic** (**silent**), do not propagate proximally and have no adverse consequences (cf. **proximal** i.e. iliofemoral thrombi which can cause pulmonary embolism [PE]). Distal (calf) thrombi usually do not require anticoagulation, but 10–20% of calf thrombi extend to the proximal veins, and then anticoagulation is indicated; this extension of the distal thrombus to the proximal veins can be detected by serial (once or twice a week) **duplex** ultrasound (US).

CANCER
Patients with cancer have a higher (about 4–6 times) risk of VTE due to several reasons, including immobilization, hypercoagulable (prothrombotic) state, surgery, **chemotherapy**, hormone therapy, use of central venous catheter (**CVC**), etc. Cancer is associated with thrombocytosis; tumours may produce **thrombin**; increased levels of **fibrinogen** and factor VIII may be present in patients with cancer.

About 20% of all new cases of VTE are in patients with cancer. Fifteen to twenty percent of patients with cancer develop VTE at some point in their illness. VTE is the second most common cause of death among cancer patients. Symptomatic VTE occurs in about 10–15% of cancer patients, but screening and autopsy studies reveal 50% prevalence of VTE in cancer patients. Patients with **unexplained** i.e. without any obvious cause VTE should be investigated for an asymptomatic cancer (Fig. C1).

Risk of VTE is higher with brain, pancreas, ovary, kidney, prostate, liver, colon, stomach and lung cancer; risk is lower in head/neck and breast cancer (though chemotherapy in these patients may increase the risk of VTE). **Hematological** cancers also carry a high risk of VTE. Major surgery in cancer caries a higher risk of VTE – calf vein thrombosis (40–80%), proximal (iliofemoral) vein thrombosis (10–20%), clinical PE (4–10%) and fatal PE (1–5%).

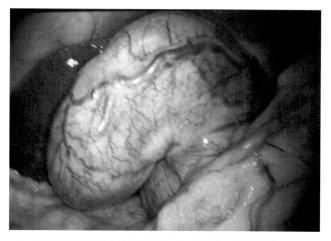

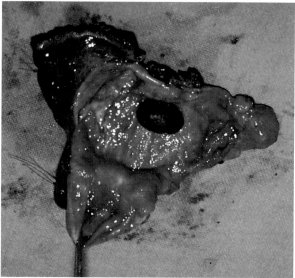

Fig. C1 This elderly gentleman presented with symptomatic bilateral deep venous thrombosis in the legs. CT abdomen was done to look for an abdominal cancer – it revealed a gallbladder mass without liver infiltration. a. Staging laparoscopy revealed a gall bladder fundus mass. Extended (radical) cholecystectomy was done. b. The specimen showed an ulcerated mass in the gallbladder fundus; a single large gallstone is also seen.

C

LMWHs are recommended for long-term (i.e. 3–6 months) treatment of VTE in cancer patients. Cancer patients are more likely to have bleeding complications on anticoagulation therapy. VTE in cancer patients delays chemotherapy/radiotherapy. Cancer patients are more likely to have recurrent VTE. VTE in a cancer patient usually indicates poor prognosis and short survival. Autopsy studies have shown that one in seven deaths in cancer patients are not because of the cancer itself but because of VTE; they could have survived if VTE were prevented.

CAPRINI
The Caprini **risk assessment** model (**RAM**) (Fig. C2) includes several factors e.g. age, obesity (body mass index [**BMI**]>25), comorbidities (e.g. chronic obstructive pulmonary disease [COPD]), venous disease, clotting disorders, **cancer**, recent (within 1 month) events, mobility, type and duration of surgery, etc., with each being assigned 1, 2, 3 or 5 points (Table C1).

The points are summed to produce a cumulative score, which classifies the patients into four risk levels viz. 0–1 (low), 2 (moderate), 3–4 (high) and 5 or more (highest). Recommendations for thromboprophylaxis are based on the score/ risk level.

Score	2	mechanical prophylaxis
	3–4	mechanical + pharmacological prophylaxis – during hospitalization
	5–8	mechanical + pharmacological prophylaxis for 7 days
	>8	mechanical + pharmacological prophylaxis for 30 days

CARDIOVASCULAR
VTE is the third most common cardiovascular disease (after coronary artery disease [CAD] and stroke) in the world.

CAT (CANCER-ASSOCIATED THROMBOSIS)
See **Cancer**.

CATHETER-DIRECTED THROMBOLYSIS (CDT)
Catheter-directed thrombolysis (CDT) is a procedure consisting of local thrombolysis through a catheter positioned either in the common iliac vein or the subclavian vein with deep venous thrombosis (DVT). This is safe, and the risk of bleeding is less. Thrombolysis can be achieved either by pharmacomechanical means or by US energy (the EkoSonic or EKOS Endo Wave Infusion Catheter System [**EKOS**]).

CAUTION
Caution is to be exercised while using thromboprophylaxis in patients with uncontrolled hypertension, gastrointestinal e.g. **peptic ulcers**, cerebrovascular accident (CVA), acute bacterial endocarditis and **renal dysfunction**.

C

DVT
Risk Assessment Form

Department :   Date:

Patient's Identification No.:   Age:

Sex: M ☐   F ☐

Height:

Weight: (kg)

Choose all that apply

A — Each Item Represents 1 Risk Factor

- Minor Surgery ☐
- Age 40-60 yrs ☐
- Pregnancy or post Partum (< 1 Month) ☐
- Varicose Veins ☐
- Inflammatory Bowel Disease ☐
- Obesity (>20% of ideal BW) ☐
- Combined Oral Contraceptives/HRT ☐

Total Tickmarks [ ] x 1

Total Score A [ ]

B — Each Item Represents 2 Risk Factors

- Age over 60 years ☐
- Malignancy ☐
- Major Surgery ☐
- Immobilising Plaster Cast ☐
- Medical or Surgical Patients Confined to Bed >72 hrs ☐
- Central Venous Access ☐

Total Tickmarks [ ] x 2

Total Score B [ ]

C — Each Item Represents 3 Risk Factors

- History of DVT / PE ☐
- Myocardial Infarction ☐
- Congestive Heart Failure ☐
- Severe Sepsis / Infection ☐
- Factor V Leiden / Activated Protein C resistance ☐
- Antithrombin III Deficiency ☐
- Proteins C and S Deficiency ☐
- Dysfibrinogenemia ☐
- Homocysteinemia ☐
- 20210A Prothrombin Mutation ☐
- Lupus Anticoagulant ☐
- Antiphospholipid Antibodies ☐
- Myeloproliferative Disorders ☐
- Disorders of Plasminogen and Plasmin Activation ☐
- Heparin-induced Thrombocytopenia ☐
- Hyperviscosity Syndromes ☐

Total Tickmarks [ ] x 3

Total Score C [ ]

D — Each Item Represents 5 Risk Factors

- Elective Major Lower Extremity Arthroplasty ☐
- Hip, Pelvis or Leg Fracture ☐
- Stroke ☐
- Multiple Trauma ☐
- Acute Spinal Cord Injury ☐

Total Tickmarks [ ] x 5

Total Score D [ ]

Total Score (A+B+C+D)= [ ]

Risk Assessment: ☐ Hightest ☐ High ☐ Moderate ☐ Low

Recommended Prophylactic Regimens for Each Risk Group

Total Score	Risk Category		Recommended Regimen			
1	Low	→	No Specific measures ☐		Early Ambulation ☐	
2	Moderate	→	LDUFH (every 12h), LMWN, IPC and GCS ☐			
3-4	High	→	LDUFH (every 8h), LMWN, and IPC ☐		GCS (+ LDUFH or LMWH) ☐	
5 or more	Highest	→	LMWH, Oral anticoagulants, Adjusted dose heparin ☐		IPC (+ LDUFH or LMWH), GCS (+LDUFH or LMWH) ☐	

LDUFH-Low dose un fractionated heparin
LMWH-Low molecular weight heparin
GCS-Graduated compression stockings
IPC-Intermittent pneumatic compression

Reason for not giving Prophylaxis _____

Compiled from Caprini JA et al, *Effective risk stratification of Surgical and Non surgical patients for venous thromboembolic disease, Semin hematol 38(Suppl 5):12-19*

Thromboprophylaxis is the Number 1 strategy to improve patient safety

Fig. C2   The Caprini risk assessment model (RAM) includes several factors, which are given 1, 2, 3 and 5 points. The points are then summed to produce a cumulative score, which classifies the patients into four risk levels.

Table C1   Caprini risk assessment model (RAM)

1 point each	2 points each
• Age 41–60 years • Minor surgery • Previous major surgery within 1 month • Varicose veins • History of (h/o) inflammatory bowel disease (IBD) • Current swollen leg • Obesity (BMI >25) • Acute myocardial infarction (MI) • Congestive heart failure (CHF) within 1 month • Sepsis within 1 month • Serious lung disease within 1 month • Abnormal lung function (COPD) • Medical patient on bed rest	• Age 60–74 years • Arthroscopic surgery • Present or previous malignancy • Major surgery (>45 minutes) • Laparoscopic surgery (>45 minutes) • Confined to bed >72 hours • Immobilizing plaster cast within 1 month • Central venous access
3 points each	5 points each
• Age >75 years • h/o DVT/PE • Family h/o VTE • Factor V Leiden • Prothrombin 20210A • Elevated serum homocysteine • Lupus anticoagulant • Anticardiolipin antibodies • Heparin-induced thrombocytopenia (HIT) • Other thrombophilia	• Major lower extremity arthroplasty • Hip, pelvis or leg fracture within 1 month • Stroke within 1 month • Multiple trauma within 1 month • Spinal cord injury (SCI)/paralysis within 1 month
	For women 1 point each
	• Oral contraceptive pills (OCPs) or hormone replacement therapy (HRT) • Pregnancy or postpartum within 1 month • h/o unexplained stillbirth, recurrent (>3) spontaneous abortion, premature birth, growth-retarded infant

CaVenT TRIAL

The Catheter-directed Venous Thrombolysis (CaVenT) trial and Acute Venous Thrombosis: Thrombus Removal with Adjunctive Catheter Directed Thrombolysis (**ATTRACT**) trial substudy provided evidence to support catheter directed thrombolysis (**CDT**) for the management of iliofemoral DVT.

C

CC (CREATININE CLEARANCE)

Caution should be exercised when using LMWHs in patients with abnormal CC due to chronic kidney disease (**CKD**). Different LMWHs have variable degrees of drug accumulation in the presence of renal impairment. Enoxaparin needs dose modification in patients with **renal dysfunction** and is contraindicated in the presence of severe renal dysfunction.

CDT

See **Catheter-directed thrombolysis (CDT)**.

CEAP CLASSIFICATION

The Clinical, Etiological, Anatomical and Pathophysiological (CEAP) classification is used to stage **varicose veins** and chronic venous insufficiency (**CVI**).

Lurie F, De Maeseneer MGR. The 2020 update of the CEAP classification: What is new? *Eur J Vasc Endovasc Surg.* 2020;59(6):859–60. doi: 10.1016/j.ejvs. 2020.04.020

CELLULITIS

The clinical features of cellulitis viz. pain, fever, swelling, tenderness, etc., may resemble those of DVT.

CENTRAL VENOUS ACCESS

Central venous access is commonly used in critically ill patients. Central venous access with a central venous catheter (**CVC**) increases the risk of DVT.

CENTRAL VENOUS CATHETER (CVC)

See **CVC**.

CEREBRAL VENOUS THROMBOSIS (CVT)

See **CVT**.

CHART

A VTE **risk assessment** (and prophylaxis) chart should be filled out for each hospitalized patient.

CHEMOTHERAPY

Cancer patients are at a high risk to develop VTE. Chemotherapy further increases the risk of VTE in patients with **cancer**. Incidence of VTE after starting chemotherapy is about 10–15% at 12 months. VTE accounts for about 10% of deaths in patients on chemotherapy. These patients should, therefore, receive long-term thromboprophylaxis.

CHEST X-RAY

The role of chest X-ray is more to exclude other chest conditions e.g. atelectasis, consolidation and pleural effusion, which can mimic PE than to diagnose PE; it has to be kept in mind, however, that all these changes can be seen in PE also. A normal chest X-ray in a patient with sudden onset of breathlessness rules out pneumonia and acute respiratory distress syndrome (**ARDS**) and strongly supports a diagnosis of PE. Chest X-ray may show evidence of oligemia or infarction in a patient with PE.

CHF (CONGESTIVE HEART FAILURE)

The **MEDENOX** study showed that **enoxaparin** prevents VTE in medical patients, including those with CHF.

Incidence of VTE (8.4% vs. 10.4%) and DVT (7.9% vs. 9.9%) was less with enoxaparin 40 mg OD (n = 239) than with unfractionated heparin (UFH) 5,000 U TID (n = 212) in patients with heart failure or severe respiratory disease.

See **ARTEMIS** also.

Samama MM, Cohen AT, Darmon JY, Desjardins L, Eldor A, Janbon C, Leizorovicz A, Nguyen H, Olsson CG, Turpie AG, Weisslinger N; Prophylaxis in Medical Patients with Enoxaparin Study Group. A comparison of enoxaparin with placebo for the prevention of venous thromboembolism in acutely ill medical patients. *N Engl J Med*. 1999;341(11):793–800. doi: 10.1056/NEJM199909093411103. PMID: 10477777

Kleber FX, Witt C, Vogel G, Koppenhagen K, Schomaker U, Flosbach CW; THE-PRINCE Study Group. Randomized comparison of enoxaparin with unfractionated heparin for the prevention of venous thromboembolism in medical patients with heart failure or severe respiratory disease. *Am Heart J*. 2003;145(4):614–21. doi: 10.1067/mhj.2003.189. PMID: 12679756

CHRONIC KIDNEY DISEASE (CKD)

See **CKD**.

CHRONIC VENOUS HYPERTENSION (CVH)

See **CVH**.

CHRONIC VENOUS INSUFFICIENCY (CVI)

See **CVI**.

CIRCUIT THROMBOSIS

Circuits of continuous renal replacement therapy (CRRT) and extracorporeal membrane oxygenation (**ECMO**) for cardiopulmonary support may develop thrombosis, which can be prevented with the use of regional and systemic anticoagulation.

CIRCUMFERENCE

Thigh and calf circumference (bilateral) should be measured daily in all patients receiving treatment for DVT to objectively monitor the progress of limb oedema.

CIRRHOSIS

Patients with cirrhosis of liver have an increased risk of bleeding with the use of thromboprophylaxis due to the associated coagulopathy.

CKD (CHRONIC KIDNEY DISEASE)

Caution should be exercised when using heparins in patients with CKD. **Creatinine clearance (CC)** is a better marker of the degree of **renal dysfunction** than serum creatinine alone.

CLINICAL DECISION RULES

Clinical decision rules are used to estimate the **probability** of DVT and PE and to stratify the patients into low, intermediate or high risk.

CLINICAL FEATURES

Pain, swelling, redness, discoloration, tenderness, fever and unilateral pitting oedema are the classical clinical features of DVT. It is important, however, to keep in mind that only one-third of patients with proven DVT have clinical symptoms and signs – the remaining two-thirds are **asymptomatic** i.e. clinically **silent**. Also, these symptoms and signs are not specific for DVT and may be present in several other conditions e.g. **cellulitis**; hence the diagnosis of DVT cannot be made merely by the presence of these clinical features and needs confirmation by investigations. Only half of those patients who are thought to have DVT on clinical grounds are found to have DVT on investigation.

CLOPIDOGREL

Antiplatelet drugs e.g. clopidogrel are useful for preventing arterial thrombosis; however, they have no role in venous thromboprophylaxis.

Platelet inhibitors such as clopidogrel should be stopped for 5–14 days if a **neuraxial** block (spinal or epidural) is planned.

CLOT STUDY

A randomized controlled trial (**RCT**) comparing LMWH (**dalteparin** 200 IU/kg once daily for 1 month followed by 150 IU/kg once daily for 5 months) alone with LMWH + **vitamin K antagonist (VKA)** therapy (dalteparin 200 IU/kg once daily for 5–7 days followed by **warfarin** for 6 months) in patients with **cancer** who had acute, symptomatic proximal **DVT**, PE or both. Symptomatic, objectively documented recurrent **VTE** was less in the dalteparin-alone group than in the warfarin group (9% vs. 17%), a relative risk reduction of 49%. There was no significant difference in major **bleeding** between the two groups.

Woodruff S, Lee AYY, Carrier M, Feugère G, Abreu P, Heissler J. Low-molecular-weight-heparin versus a coumarin for the prevention of recurrent venous thromboembolism in high- and low-risk patients with active cancer: a post hoc analysis of the CLOT Study. *J Thromb Thrombolysis.* 2019;47(4):495–504. doi: 10.1007/s11239-019-01833-w. PMID: 30859370

CMC (CHRISTIAN MEDICAL COLLEGE)

VTE was present in 17 per 10,000 admissions at the Christian Medical College (CMC), Vellore India. The most common risk factors for VTE were **cancer** (present in 31% of cases) and postoperative status (present in 30% of cases). Mortality of PE was 13%.

Lee AD, Stephen E, Agarwal S, Premkumar P. Venous thromboembolism in India. *Eur J Vasc Endovasc Surg.* 2009;37(4):482–85. doi: 10.1016/j.ejvs.2008.11.031. Epub 2009 Feb 8. PMID: 19208449

COAGULATION CASCADE

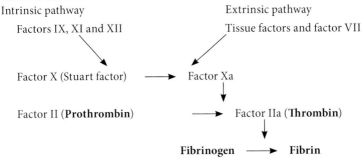

- UFH acts on factors Xa and IIa and on factors XIIa, XIa and IXa.
- **Warfarin** acts on factors Xa and IIa and on factors VIIa and IXa.
- LMWHs acts on factors Xa and IIa.
- **Fondaparinux** acts on factor Xa alone.

COAGULATION PROFILE

A complete coagulation profile includes platelet count, platelet aggregation, bleeding time, clotting time, activated clotting time (**ACT**), prothrombin time (**PT**), international normalized ratio (**INR**) and activated partial thromboplastin time (**aPTT**).

COCHRANE DATABASE

The Cochrane Database is a collection of high-quality evidence to inform and guide healthcare decision-making.

Kirkilesis G, Kakkos SK, Bicknell C, Salim S, Kakavia K. Treatment of distal deep vein thrombosis. *Cochrane Database Syst Rev.* 2020;4(4):CD013422. Published 2020 Apr 9. Doi :10.1002/14651858.CD013422.pub2

COLOUR DOPPLER

Colour Doppler measures the blood flow in the veins – no or limited blood flow is seen in a thrombosed vein in DVT. Colour Doppler is more sensitive in detecting DVT in **symptomatic** (sensitivity 90%) than in **asymptomatic** (**silent**) (sensitivity 60%) cases.

See **Doppler** also.

COMBINATION

Pooled results of randomized controlled trials (**RCTs**) show that a combination of mechanical methods e.g. graduated compression stockings (**GCS**) with pharmacological prophylaxis is better than GCS alone.

Amaragiri SV, Lees TA. Elastic compression stockings for prevention of deep vein thrombosis. *Cochrane Database Syst Rev.* 2000;(3):CD001484. doi: 10.1002/14651858.CD001484. PMID: 10908501

COMORBIDITIES

Comorbidities e.g. acute myocardial infarction (**MI**), congestive heart failure (**CHF**) and chronic obstructive pulmonary disease (COPD) are risk factors for VTE.

COMPRESSION US (ULTRASONOGRAPHY)

A normal (patent) vein is totally compressible. A thrombosed (obliterated) vein is incompressible i.e. cannot be compressed completely on pressure of the US probe.

COMPUTER-BASED

A computer-based prompt can alert the physician to prescribe thromboprophylaxis unless 'no-prophylaxis' is documented for a given patient.

COMPUTER (ELECTRONIC) ALERT

A computer-based (electronic) alert programme has been described to encourage the use of VTE prophylaxis.

Kucher N, Koo S, Quiroz R, Cooper JM, Paterno MD, Soukonnikov B, Goldhaber SZ. Electronic alerts to prevent venous thromboembolism among hospitalized patients. *N Engl J Med.* 2005;352(10):969–77. doi: 10.1056/NEJMoa041533. PMID: 15758007

CONSENSUS STATEMENTS

Consensus encourage and **guidelines** of several international societies and organizations strongly recommend thromboprophylaxis in indicated patients.

CONSEQUENCE

PE is a dangerous and **fatal** consequence of DVT and may occur in 20–50% of cases of DVT.

See **Sequelae** also.

CONTRAINDICATIONS

Thromboprophylaxis is contraindicated in patients with active and uncontrolled bleeding, those who are at high risk for bleeding e.g. active **peptic ulcer** disease (PUD), coagulopathy (**INR** >1.5), thrombocytopenia (platelets <50,000), recent haemorrhagic **stroke**, heparin-induced thrombocytopenia (**HIT**), and hypersensitivity to **heparins**.

Thrombotherapy is contraindicated in patients with intracranial tumour, intracranial haemorrhage and **stroke** within 3 months. Recent eye and intracranial surgery are also contraindications for the use of pharmacological thromboprophylaxis.

CONTRAST US (ULTRASONOGRAPHY)

Contrast US, using intravenous contrast in the form of microbubbles of gas, is better than conventional US for the diagnosis of DVT.

COST

The annual healthcare burden of VTE is about $1.5 billion in the United States. The cost of managing each episode of DVT is about $10,000 in the United States. The estimated costs to avoid a VTE event in medical patients (e.g. congestive heart failure, acute respiratory failure and acute infection) are about $1,100–1,500.

In another study (McGarry. *Am J Manag Care* 2004), the cost of avoiding one VTE death was $9,000.

Pechevis (*Value Health* 2000) calculated a cost of about Euro 8,000 to prevent one death from VTE. VTE prophylaxis (with **enoxaparin**) accounted for only 1.2–2.4% of the total costs for the admission (de Lissovoy. *Am J Manag Care* 2002).

LMWHs are more expensive than UFH but have the advantages of outpatient treatment, once-daily (cf. twice or thrice daily for UFH) administration and less risk of heparin-induced thrombocytopenia (**HIT**) and **osteoporosis** (on long-term administration). They are thus cost-saving and **cost-effective**.

de Lissovoy G, Subedi P. Economic evaluation of enoxaparin as prophylaxis against venous thromboembolism in seriously ill medical patients: a US perspective. *Am J Manag Care.* 2002;8(12):1082–88. PMID: 12500884

McGarry LJ, Thompson D, Weinstein MC, Goldhaber SZ. Cost effectiveness of thromboprophylaxis with a low-molecular-weight heparin versus unfractionated heparin in acutely ill medical inpatients. *Am J Manag Care.* 2004;10(9):632–42. PMID: 15515996

Pechevis M, Detournay B, Pribil C, Fagnani F, Chalanson G. Economic evaluation of enoxaparin vs. placebo for the prevention of venous thromboembolism in acutely ill medical patients. *Value Health.* 2000;3(6):389–96. doi: 10.1046/j.1524-4733.2000.36008.x. PMID: 16464198

COST-EFFECTIVE

In the first instance, it may appear that the use of VTE prophylaxis will increase the **cost** of treatment of the patients, but in the final analysis, VTE prophylaxis is cost-effective – at least in high-risk patients, because the occurrence of DVT and PE in the absence of prophylaxis leads to prolonged hospitalization for investigations and management and increases the overall costs of treatment.

CORONA-VTE NET

COVID-19 Registry to Assess Frequency, Risk Factors, Management, and Outcomes of Arterial and Venous Thromboembolic Complications

This is a proposed electronic health record (EHR)–guided, 10,000-patient, retrospective observational cohort study to assess VTE incidence, risk factors, prevention and management patterns and thrombotic outcomes in patients with **COVID-19** infection. A 5,000-patient cohort will be enrolled within the Massachusetts General Brigham Network in Boston Massachusetts USA, with 1,000 patients each at five additional sites.

https://clinicaltrials.gov/ct2/show/NCT04535128

COVAC TP

COVID-19 Anticoagulation in Children – Thromboprophylaxis (COVAC-TP) Trial

A proposed study to evaluate the safety, dose requirements and exploratory efficacy of twice-daily subcutaneous **enoxaparin** as VTE prophylaxis in children (birth to 18 years) hospitalized with signs and/or symptoms of SARS-CoV-2 infection (i.e. COVID-19).

https://clinicaltrials.gov/ct2/show/NCT04354155

COVID-19

Coronavirus disease (COVID) emerged as a major global health problem in 2020 and became a pandemic. Much of the morbidity and mortality of COVID is attributed to adult respiratory distress syndrome (ARDS), but COVID is a hypercoagulable thromboinflammatory state, having endothelial dysfunction and coagulopathy; thrombosis is venous in 80–90% and arterial in 10–20% of patients with COVID-19. Abnormal coagulation profile, especially markedly elevated **D-dimer** and fibrin degradation products (FDP), have been associated with a poor prognosis in COVID-19 infection. Anticoagulation is an important component of the treatment bundle of COVID.

CPB

Massive PE may require surgical intervention. Cardiopulmonary bypass (CPB) is required for the surgical management of PE.

CREATININE CLEARANCE (CC)

See **CC**.

CREPE BANDAGE

A crepe bandage (Fig C3), while useful in the management of **varicose veins**, does not offer any protection against DVT. Graduated compression stockings (**GCS**) should be used instead.

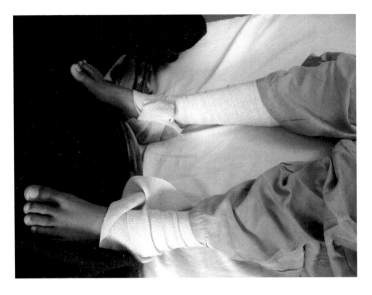

Fig. C3   A crepe bandage applies unequal nongradient pressure and is not recommended for the management of DVT.

CTA (CT ANGIOGRAPHY)
See **CTPA**.

CTPA (CT PULMONARY ANGIOGRAPHY)
CT pulmonary angiography (CTPA) (Fig. C4) is replacing conventional angiography as the standard investigation for the diagnosis of PE (Fig. C5); a normal CTPA virtually rules out PE.

CTPH (CHRONIC THROMBOEMBOLIC PULMONARY HYPERTENSION)
About 5% of patients with PE go on to develop chronic thromboembolic pulmonary hypertension (CTPH).

CT PULMONARY ANGIOGRAPHY (CTPA)
See **CTPA**.

CUMULATIVE
Risk factors for VTE have a cumulative (additive) effect. The presence of multiple risk factors increases the risk of VTE manyfold.

C

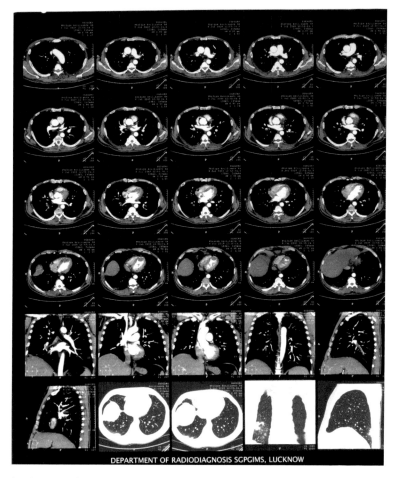

DEPARTMENT OF RADIODIAGNOSIS SGPGIMS, LUCKNOW

Fig. C4 CT pulmonary angiography (CTPA) is the investigation of choice for the diagnosis of pulmonary embolism.

CURVE

The CURVE study included a chart audit in 29 Canadian hospitals – 90% of acutely ill medical patients had an indication for thromboprophylaxis, but only 16% received adequate prophylaxis.

Kahn SR, Panju A, Geerts W, Pineo GF, Desjardins L, Turpie AG, Glezer S, Thabane L, Sebaldt RJ; CURVE study investigators. Multicenter evaluation of the use of venous thromboembolism prophylaxis in acutely ill medical patients in Canada. *Thromb Res.* 2007;119(2):145–55. doi: 10.1016/j. thromres.2006.01.011. Epub 2006 Mar 3. PMID: 16516275

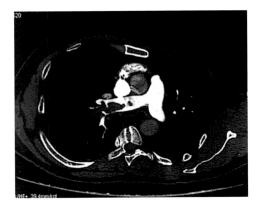

Fig. C5　CT pulmonary angiography (CTPA) shows a large embolus in the right pulmonary artery and its posterior branch. (Image courtesy of Dr Shivani Rao, Indira Gandhi Medical College, Shimla.)

CUS (COMPRESSION US)
Pressure of the US probe will compress a normal (patent) vein but not a thrombosed (obliterated) vein in DVT.

CVC (CENTRAL VENOUS CATHETER)
Long-term use of a CVC (Fig. C6) is associated with a higher risk of DVT; prophylaxis to reduce this risk, however, is controversial and is not recommended.

CVH (CHRONIC VENOUS HYPERTENSION)
Long-standing DVT in the lower limb causes destruction of the valves in the veins leading to chronic venous hypertension (CVH). This causes painful and tender swelling of the leg (Fig. C7a), varicosities (Fig. C7b) and skin changes e.g. **pigmentation** (Fig. C7c), **ulcers** (Fig. C7d), etc. CVH is the most common cause of leg ulcers.

CVI (CHRONIC VENOUS INSUFFICIENCY)
CVI is one of the disabling **sequelae** of DVT – it results in chronic oedema, **cellulitis**, **pigmentation** and recurrent venous **ulcers**.

CVT (CEREBRAL VENOUS THROMBOSIS)
Cerebral venous thrombosis (CVT) occurs in puerperal women. It is more common in India than in the West. This is due to a reversible **hypercoagulable** state in the postpartum period and requires therapeutic anticoagulation for 2–3 weeks.

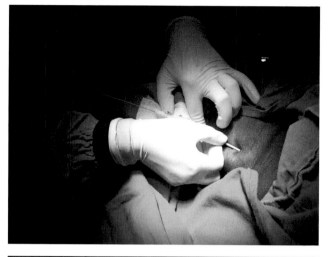

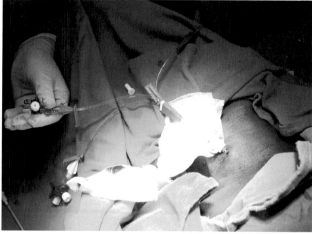

Fig. C6   a and b. Long-term use of central venous catheter (CVC) is a risk factor for venous thromboembolism (VTE).

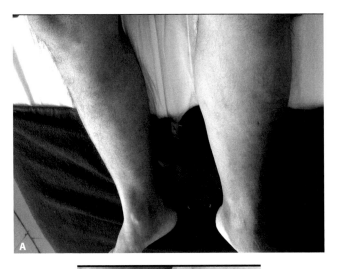

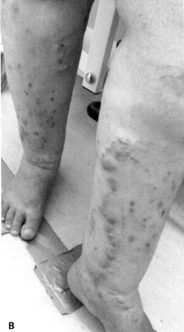

Fig. C7 Chronic venous hypertension (CVH) caused by deep venous thrombosis (DVT) resulting in a. oedema, b. varicosities, c. pigmentation and d. ulceration. (*Continued*)

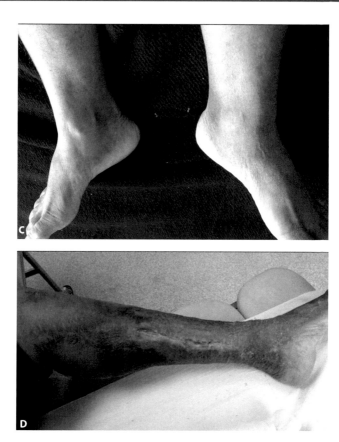

Fig. C7 (Cont.) Chronic venous hypertension (CVH) caused by deep venous thrombosis (DVT) resulting in a. oedema, b. varicosities, c. pigmentation and d. ulceration.

D

DABIGATRAN

- Dabigatran is a direct oral anticoagulant (**DOAC**); it is an anti-IIa agent - a direct thrombin inhibitor (**DTI**).
- Dabigatran is indicated for the prophylaxis of deep venous thrombosis (DVT) and pulmonary embolism (PE) following hip replacement surgery only.
- Dose for prophylaxis – 110 mg PO on day 1 (after surgery) and then 220 mg PO daily for 28–35 days
- Dose for treatment – 150 mg BID after low-molecular-weight heparin (LMWH) for the initial 5–10 days

Idarucizumab can neutralize the effects of dabigatran.

DALTEPARIN

Dalteparin is one of the LMWHs. Molecular weight is 5,700 Da; half-life is 2 hours and **anti-Xa/anti-IIa** ratio is 2.7:1.

The dose for prophylaxis of VTE is 2,500 IU SC OD started 1–2 hours preoperatively in low- and moderate-risk patients and 5,000 IU SC OD started 8–12 hours preoperatively in high-risk surgical patients.

The dose for treatment of VTE is 200 IU per kg SC OD or 100 IU per kg SC BID.

DANAPAROID

Danaparoid is a heparin derivative (**heparinoid**) – a specific factor Xa inhibitor. It may be useful in patients with heparin-induced thrombocytopenia (**HIT**).

DASH

The DASH (**D-dimer, age, sex, hormone** use) rule is used to decide about the continuation or stoppage of anticoagulation in a patient with VTE after 3–6 months.

Abnormal D-dimer (measured 1 month after stopping anticoagulation) +2, age <50 years +1, male sex +1, hormone use in female –2

0 or 1: annual risk of recurrent VTE is 3%; anticoagulation may be discontinued.

2 or more: annual risk of recurrent VTE is 9%; anticoagulation may be continued.

DAY-CARE SURGERY

The risk of DVT in patients undergoing day-care surgery is very low. Recommendations for thromboprophylaxis depend on the procedure-related and personal **risk factors**:

1. Low-risk procedure without additional risk factors: General measures (i.e. early **ambulation**, optimal hydration) of thromboprophylaxis
2. Low-risk procedure with additional risk factors or high-risk procedure without additional risk factors: Pharmacological prophylaxis with LMWHs

Pharmacological prophylaxis can be limited to hospitalization or may extend to 7 days or 4 weeks, depending on the risk calculation.

Venclauskas L, Llau JV, Jenny JY, Kjaersgaard-Andersen P, Jans Ø; ESA VTE Guidelines Task Force. European guidelines on perioperative venous thromboembolism prophylaxis: Day surgery and fast-track surgery. *Eur J Anaesthesiol.* 2018;35(2):134–38. doi: 10.1097/EJA.0000000000000706

D-DIMER

D-dimer (so called because it contains two cross-linked fragments of fibrin protein) measures fibrin degradation products (FDPs) in plasma and is an indicator of ongoing fibrinolysis. It is useful for **screening** for VTE. At a cutoff of 500 micro g/L, it has high (90–95%) sensitivity, which means that a negative D-dimer virtually excludes the diagnosis of VTE, especially if the clinical suspicion is low. Negative D-dimer in a low-risk patient indicates 99% probability that there is no DVT. But D-dimer has low (30–40%) specificity, which means that a positive D-dimer does not necessarily mean the presence of DVT, as it may be positive due to infection/sepsis, active bleeding, myocardial infarction (**MI**), **pregnancy**, **cancer**, **trauma** and in the postoperative period. But positive D-dimer in a high-risk patient indicates a 75% chance of DVT. It thus has a high negative predictive value (NPV) and low positive predictive value (PPV). Both qualitative and quantitative (enzyme-linked immunosorbent assay [ELISA] or turbidimetric) assays can be done for D-dimer.

D-dimer should be used in low- or intermediate-risk (pretest probability [**PTP**]) cases only, not in high-risk cases where imaging (**Doppler** ultrasound [US] for DVT and CT pulmonary angiography [**CTPA**] for PE) should be done.

DEATHS

About 300,000 deaths occur due to PE every year in the United States (population 300 million). In the European Union (population 500 million), VTE is estimated to cause about 500,000 deaths every year. This is more than the deaths due to acquired immunodeficiency syndrome (AIDS), breast cancer and road accidents combined. In the UK, PE is responsible for 3% of surgical and 10% of all hospital deaths. About 1% of all hospital admissions die from PE. PE is the third most common cause of death in hospitalized patients in the United States. Ten percent of patients with PE die within 1 hour – the window for diagnosis and treatment is thus very narrow. Six percent of patients with DVT and 12% with PE die within 1 month of the diagnosis.

In the West, PE is a common cause of death of puerperal women and postsurgical patients. In a study of 51,645 hospitalized patients in USA, PE was present in 1% of patients. It was the cause of death or contributed to death in 37% of patients who died (Stein. *Chest* 1995).

Stein PD, Henry JW. Prevalence of acute pulmonary embolism among patients in a general hospital and at autopsy. *Chest*. 1995;108(4):978–81. doi: 10.1378/chest.108.4.978. PMID: 7555172

DEEP VEINS
Deep veins of the lower extremity include the common femoral vein (CFV), deep and superficial femoral veins, popliteal vein, anterior and posterior tibial veins and the peroneal vein.

Deep veins of the upper extremity include the subclavian vein, axillary vein, brachial vein, radial vein, ulnar vein and the interosseus vein.

DEFAULT PROPHYLAXIS
There are several strategies for using VTE prophylaxis. Default prophylaxis is one of the strategies in which VTE prophylaxis is given to all patients; it is omitted in patients at low risk only.

DEFICIENCY
Patients with deficiency of natural anticoagulants such as **antithrombin 3** and **protein C and S** have an irreversible hypercoagulable state, and some of these patients may require lifelong anticoagulation to prevent VTE.

DEHYDRATION
Dehydration increases the risk of DVT by causing venous stasis. Patients at risk of DVT should be kept well hydrated.

DE NOVO
Idiopathic or **unprovoked** DVT.

DEXTRAN
Low (40, 70) molecular weight dextran has a limited and doubtful role in anticoagulation prophylaxis and treatment.

DIAGNOSIS
It is difficult to diagnose DVT because majority of the cases are **asymptomatic** (**silent**) and the diagnosis is not even suspected; even when DVT is suspected, it is difficult to prove by investigations. Only 30% of DVT is diagnosed antemortem. In 70–80% of patients who die of PE, the diagnosis of PE is not even considered before death.

See **Autopsy** also.

DIFFERENTIAL DIAGNOSIS

1. The differential diagnosis of DVT includes **cellulitis**, lymphedema, chronic venous insufficiency (**CVI**), etc.

2. Symptoms and signs of PE resemble those of the more common postoperative complications e.g. chest infection, adult respiratory distress syndrome (**ARDS**), myocardial infarction (**MI**), etc. Pneumonia, bronchitis, acute exacerbation of chronic obstructive airways disease (COAD), pleuritis, costochondritis, congestive heart failure (**CHF**), pulmonary oedema and pericarditis can also mimic PE.

DIALYSIS

Dialysis (Fig. D1) patients are at increased risk of VTE.

DIPYRIDAMOLE

Dipyridamole is an **antiplatelet** drug which was earlier used in patients with replaced heart valves and coronary artery disease (CAD). If it is being used, it should be stopped 48 hours before surgery.

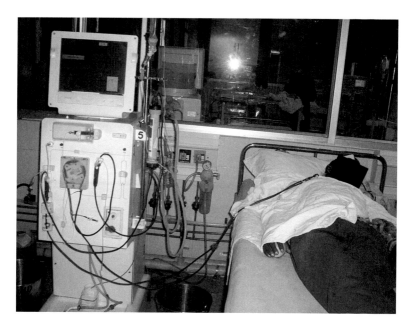

Fig. D1   Patients on dialysis are at a higher risk to develop venous thromboembolism.

D

DIRECT STUDY

In 120 critically ill patients, all with **creatinine clearance (CC)** <30 mL/minute, there was no bioaccumulation of **dalteparin** when used for prophylaxis in a dose of 5,000 U OD.

Douketis J, Cook D, Meade M, Guyatt G, Geerts W, Skrobik Y, Albert M, Granton J, Hébert P, Pagliarello G, Marshall J, Fowler R, Freitag A, Rabbat C, Anderson D, Zytaruk N, Heels-Ansdell D, Crowther M; Canadian Critical Care Trials Group. Prophylaxis against deep vein thrombosis in critically ill patients with severe renal insufficiency with the low-molecular-weight heparin dalteparin: An assessment of safety and pharmacodynamics: The DIRECT study. *Arch Intern Med.* 2008;168(16):1805–12. doi: 10.1001/archinte.168.16.1805. PMID: 18779469

DISCHARGE

A large number of VTEs occur after the discharge of the patient from the hospital, hence the need for **extended prophylaxis.** This is true for patients who have undergone major **orthopaedic surgery** or those with **cancer**.

DOAC (DIRECT ORAL ANTICOAGULANTS)

DOACs include **dabigatran** a direct thrombin inhibitor [**DTI**] and **apixaban**, **rivaroxaban** and **edoxaban** (anti–factor Xa). They have similar efficacy and side effect profile compared to warfarin. They are now being increasingly used for **extended** post-discharge prophylaxis.

Advantages of DOACs include oral administration, limited interaction with other drugs and food (cf. vitamin K antagonists [**VKA**s]), no need to monitor and easier to manage except in patients with **renal dysfunction**. They are usually preferred over VKAs but are expensive. **Antidote**s are now available (especially against dabigatran) in case reversal of their effect is required to stop bleeding.

See **NOA** or **NOAC** also.

DOPPLER US

Doppler US is the most preferred investigation for **screening** and diagnosis of DVT, as it is accurate and noninvasive and hence repeatable. A 4 MHz probe is used for the deep veins and 8 MHz for the superficial veins. Normal venous flow is phasic with respiration; continuous flow without phasic pattern suggests DVT. Obliterated lumen, lack of flow and lack of compressibility are US features of DVT. Doppler is highly sensitive and specific for proximal DVT; for distal (calf) DVT, though, specificity is high i.e. if Doppler shows a thrombus it is very likely to be present but sensitivity is low i.e. not all thrombi are seen on Doppler.

DOSE

Two dose regimens are used for pharmacological prophylaxis: fixed-dose and (body) weight-based dose.

DOSE FOR PROPHYLAXIS

	Moderate risk	High risk
UFH	5,000 IU SC BID	5,000 IU SC TID
LMWH	(2 hours before surgery)	(10–12 hours before surgery)
Bemiparin	2,500 IU SC OD	3,500 IU SC OD
Dalteparin	2,500 IU SC OD	5,000 IU SC OD
Enoxaparin	20 mg SC OD	40 mg SC OD
Nadroparin	2,850 IU SC OD	3,800 IU SC OD
Parnaparin	3,200 IU SC OD	4,250 IU SC OD
Tinzaparin	3,500 U SC OD	50 U/kg SC OD
Fondaparinux	2.5 mg SC OD starting at least 6 hours after surgery	
Warfarin	1 mg oral daily	

DOSE RESPONSE

LMWH has a much more predictable dose response than unfractionated heparin (UFH). This is the reason why activated partial thromboplastin time (**aPTT**) monitoring, which is essential for UFH, is not required for LMWH.

DOSE FOR TREATMENT

UFH	Initial IV bolus 80 U/kg followed by IV infusion 18 U/kg/hour – guided by **aPTT**
Bemiparin	115 IU/kg OD
Dalteparin	100 IU/kg SC BID or 200 IU/kg SC OD
Enoxaparin	1 mg/kg SC BID or 1.5 mg/kg SC OD
Nadroparin	4,100 IU BID
Parnaparin	4,250 IU SC OD
Tinzaparin	175 U/kg OD
Fondaparinux	2.5–5.0 mg SC OD for body weight <50 kg
	5.0–7.5 mg SC OD for body weight 50–100 kg
	7.5–10.0 mg SC OD for body weight >100 kg
Warfarin	5–10 mg PO daily should be started within 72 hours of heparinization, and heparin can be discontinued when international normalized ratio (**INR**) = 2.0–3.0 for at least 24 hours

DOUBLE-BLIND TRIALS

Where neither the patients nor the administering and evaluating teams know which drug is being administered to which patient. This is the best way to eliminate any evaluation bias.

DRUG INTERACTIONS

Warfarin interacts with several drugs e.g. **aspirin**, acetaminophen, amiodarone, antacids, several antibiotics, antifungals, ibuprofen, which may potentiate its anticoagulant property and cause bleeding. In India, where **tuberculosis** is still common, antitubercular drugs isoniazid and rifampicin interact with warfarin and enhance its anticoagulant effect. Drug charts of patients on warfarin should be carefully reviewed for any possible drug interaction.

See **Food interactions** also.

DTI (DIRECT THROMBIN INHIBITOR)

Antithrombin (**anti-IIa**) agents e.g. **argatroban, dabigatran, melagatran**.

DUPLEX

Duplex US is the first investigation of choice for a diagnosis of DVT, as it is easily available, inexpensive and noninvasive. Absence of flow or decreased flow and noncompressibility of the vein indicate thrombosis. The major disadvantage is that it is highly operator dependent i.e. requires skill and experience.

DURATION FOR PROPHYLAXIS

General surgery patients with a high risk of VTE should receive prophylaxis for at least 7–10 days. Prophylaxis should be given until the patient is ambulant or is discharged from the hospital.

Prophylaxis in medical patients with restricted mobility should be given for at least 7–14 days.

Extended prophylaxis (4–5 weeks) is required after major **orthopaedic surgery,** in patients with **cancer** and in those with **de novo (idiopathic)** DVT.

DURATION FOR TREATMENT

The first episode of VTE with a known transient or reversible cause (e.g. trauma, immobilization, surgery) should be treated for 6 weeks to 3 months; proximal (thigh) DVT needs longer (3 months) treatment than distal (calf) DVT (6 weeks).

Symptomatic DVT: 6 months

DVT with **cancer**: 3–6 months or as long as the cancer is active, whichever is longer; safety of LMWH beyond 6 months, however, is under investigation

Idiopathic DVT: 6–12 months

Recurrent (two or more episodes) DVT, **thrombophilia**: Lifelong

D

DURATION OF SURGERY

Duration of surgery decides the risk of VTE. Surgery >30 minutes under general anaesthesia (GA) is a risk factor for VTE.

DVT (DEEP VENOUS THROMBOSIS)

DVT occurs commonly in the lower limb. **Upper limb**, **mesenteric/portal** and pelvic veins may rarely be involved. A painful, red, swollen leg is the classical clinical picture of DVT. It must, however, be remembered that DVT is often clinically **asymptomatic (silent)**.

DVT FREE

VTE can occur in any and every setting. A review of 5,451 patients with DVT/PE (diagnosed on US) in hospitals in the United States revealed that half of these patients were outpatients (i.e. not hospitalized), while the remaining half were inpatients (i.e. hospitalized). Out of those who were hospitalized, only 22% were admitted in the intensive care unit (ICU) and as many as 78% were admitted on non-ICU beds. Only 42% of these 5,451 patients had received prophylaxis (only 32% in medical patients).

Goldhaber SZ, Tapson VF; DVT FREE Steering Committee. A prospective registry of 5,451 patients with ultrasound-confirmed deep vein thrombosis. *Am J Cardiol.* 2004;93(2):259–62. doi: 10.1016/j.amjcard.2003.09.057. PMID: 14715365

E

EAU (EUROPEAN ASSOCIATION OF UROLOGY)
https://uroweb.org/guideline/thromboprophylaxis/

ECG
The role of electrocardiogram (ECG) is more to exclude myocardial infarction (**MI**) which can mimic PE than to diagnose pulmonary embolism (PE). The ECG in PE shows sinus tachycardia, T-wave inversion in V1–V4, ST-segment depression in V5–V6 and right ventricular strain pattern; right bundle branch block (RBBB) may be present. Absence of these changes, however, does not rule out PE, as these ECG changes are present in less than one-quarter of cases with PE. ECG is more useful to diagnose cardiac conditions e.g. **MI** that mimic PE.

ECHO (ECHOCARDIOGRAPHY)
Echocardiography (echo) is more useful to exclude other conditions e.g. **MI** and cardiac tamponade which can mimic PE than to diagnose PE. Echocardiography (transthoracic and transoesophageal) reveals pulmonary arterial hypertension (**PAH**) and right ventricle dysfunction and dilatation in PE – this indicates a very poor prognosis of PE. Transoesophageal echo may also show the embolus itself in the pulmonary artery. In a patient with PE, echo reveals an enlarged right atrium and right ventricle and a collapsed left atrium and left ventricle. Normal right ventricular (RV) function on echo, however, does not rule out PE.

ECMO (EXTRACORPOREAL MEMBRANE OXYGENATION)
A circuit of extracorporeal membrane oxygenation (ECMO) for cardiopulmonary support may develop thrombosis, which can be prevented with the use of regional and systemic anticoagulation.

EDOXABAN
An oral **anti-Xa** anticoagulant.
See **DOAC** also.

EFFECTIVE
Thromboprophylaxis is effective. A meta-analysis of 70 randomized controlled trials (**RCTs**) including 16,000 patients showed that prophylaxis prevented two-thirds of deep venous thrombosis (DVT) and one-half of pulmonary embolism (PE) with no or little increase in significant bleeding.

E

Collins R, Scrimgeour A, Yusuf S, Peto R. Reduction in fatal pulmonary embolism and venous thrombosis by perioperative administration of subcutaneous heparin. Overview of results of randomized trials in general, orthopedic, and urologic surgery. *N Engl J Med.* 1988;318(18):1162–73. doi: 10.1056/NEJM198805053181805

E HIT

Endovenous heat-induced thrombosis (E HIT) occurs when endovenous thermal ablation done for **varicose veins** leads to DVT if the tip of the catheter is very near the saphenofemoral junction.

EKOS

Catheter-directed thrombolysis (**CDT**) using thrombolytic agents with acoustic streaming and ultrasound energy using the EkoSonic or EKOS Endo Wave Infusion Catheter System (EKOS Corporation, Bothell, WA, USA). Advantages include use of lower dose for shorter time of thrombolytic agents.

ELASTIC COMPRESSION STOCKINGS (ECS)

Elastic compression stockings (ECS) reduce the risk of post-thrombotic syndrome (**PTS**) after DVT. To be effective, however, they have to be used for a minimum of 1 year after an attack of DVT.

See **GCS, GECS** also.

ELECTRONIC ALERTS

Electronic alerts to physicians encouraged the use of venous thromboembolism (VTE) prophylaxis and reduced the incidence of VTE.

ELDERLY

Patients older than 40 years are at a higher risk of developing VTE.

Patients older than 75 years may have renal function impairment resulting in reduced elimination and, therefore, increased risk of bleeding with the use of **heparins**. **Dalteparin** has been approved by the U.S. Food and Drug Administration (FDA) to be safe and effective in elderly persons.

EMBOLECTOMY

Surgical embolectomy may be required for a large (**massive**) PE if medical treatment does not show response in 1–2 hours. The **window** of time between the diagnosis and management in PE, however, is very narrow.

See **Thrombectomy, Surgical** also.

EMBOLUS

An embolus is a detached piece of **thrombus** which lodges in a vessel at a distant site – it could be arterial or venous.

E

ENDORSE

Epidemiologic International Day for Evaluation of Patients at Risk for VTE in Acute Hospital Care Setting – a multinational, observational, cross-sectional survey to assess the prevalence of VTE risk in an acute hospital care setting and to determine the proportion of at-risk patients receiving prophylaxis.

In 32 countries, 358 hospitals and 68,183 patients – 37,356 (55%) medical and 30,827 (45%) surgical – 52% (42% medical and 64% surgical) of patients were found to be at risk of VTE. Of those at risk, only 50% (40% medical and 59% surgical) of patients received adequate VTE prophylaxis.

India contributed 2,058 patients (948, 46% medical and 1,110, 54% surgical), and 54% (45% medical and 61% surgical) of patients in India were found to be at risk of VTE; only 17% (22% medical and 19% surgical) of patients who were at risk of VTE received any VTE prophylaxis. Only 19% of medical and 16% of surgical patients at risk of VTE received appropriate i.e. American College of Clinical Pharmacy (**ACCP**) – recommended VTE prophylaxis.

A large proportion of hospitalized patients was at risk for VTE, but the rate of appropriate prophylaxis was low. The study reinforced the rationale for the use of hospital-wide strategies to assess the patients for their risk of VTE and to ensure that patients who are at risk receive appropriate prophylaxis.

Cohen AT, Tapson VF, Bergmann JF, Goldhaber SZ, Kakkar AK, Deslandes B, Huang W, Zayaruzny M, Emery L, Anderson FA Jr; ENDORSE Investigators. Venous thromboembolism risk and prophylaxis in the acute hospital care setting (ENDORSE study): A multinational cross-sectional study. *Lancet*. 2008;371(9610):387–94. doi: 10.1016/S0140-6736(08)60202-0. PMID: 18242412

ENDOVASCULAR

An endovascular approach is a less invasive option to surgical **thrombectomy**. It involves **thrombolysis** including catheter directed thrombolysis (**CDT**), **balloon dilatation** and **stent** placement.

ENOXACAN II TRIAL

Extended (up to 3 weeks) secondary prophylaxis in patients with existing DVT with a low-molecular-weight heparin (LMWH) (**enoxaparin**) 40 mg once-daily (OD) after major surgery for abdominal or pelvic **cancer** reduced the risk of VTE; DVT reduced from 12% to 5%.

Bergqvist D, Agnelli G, Cohen AT, Eldor A, Nilsson PE, Le Moigne-Amrani A, Dietrich-Neto F; ENOXACAN II Investigators. Duration of prophylaxis against venous thromboembolism with enoxaparin after surgery for cancer. *N Engl J Med*. 2002;346(13):975–80.

ENOXAPARIN

Enoxaparin is one of the LMWHs. Molecular weight is 4,500 Da; half-life is 4–5 hours and **anti-Xa** to **anti-IIa** ratio is 3.8:1. It has several advantages over unfractionated heparin (UFH): less major bleeding, fewer adverse events, once-daily (OD) dose (cf. twice or thrice daily for UFH) and requires no monitoring.

The dose for prophylaxis of VTE is 20 mg SC OD in moderate-risk patients and 40 mg SC OD in high-risk patients, or 30 mg SC BID started 1–2 hours pre-operatively in low- or moderate-risk surgical patients and 12 hours preoperatively in high-risk surgical patients.

The dose for the treatment of VTE is 1 mg/kg SC BID or 1.5 mg/kg SC OD.

EPHESUS

In 2,309 patients undergoing hip replacement therapy, **fondaparinux** was better than **enoxaparin** (VTE 37/908, 4% vs. 85/919, 9%).

Lassen MR, Bauer KA, Eriksson BI, Turpie AG; European Pentasaccharide Elective Surgery Study (EPHESUS) Steering Committee. Postoperative fondaparinux versus preoperative enoxaparin for prevention of venous thromboembolism in elective hip-replacement surgery: A randomised double-blind comparison. *Lancet.* 2002;359(9319):1715–20. doi: 10.1016/S0140-6736(02)08652-X. PMID: 12049858

EPIDURAL ANAESTHESIA
See **Neuraxial anaesthesia**

ESMO (EUROPEAN SOCIETY OF MEDICAL ONCOLOGY)
https://www.esmo.org/guidelines/supportive-and-palliative-care/venous-thromboembolism-vte-in-cancer-patients

E THROMBOSIS
Persons who sit at a computer for a long time are more likely to develop DVT.

EU (EUROPEAN UNION)
A reported 500,000 deaths occur in the European Union (EU) (population 500 million) due to VTE every year.

EUROPEAN ASSOCIATION OF UROLOGY (EAU)
See **EAU**.

EUROPEAN SOCIETY OF MEDICAL ONCOLOGY (ESMO)
See **ESMO**.

EVIDENCE

In spite of strong evidence in favour of the usefulness of VTE prophylaxis, several surveys from around the world show that prophylaxis is not used to the extent that it should be.

EXCLAIM

Randomized, parallel, placebo-controlled trial conducted at 370 sites in 20 countries across North and South America, Europe and Asia investigating **enoxaparin**, 40 mg/day subcutaneously (2,975 patients) or placebo (2,988 patients) for 28 +/- 4 days after receiving open-label enoxaparin for an initial 10 +/- 4 days. Extended-duration enoxaparin reduced VTE incidence compared with placebo (2.5% vs. 4%) but increased major bleeding events (0.8% vs. 0.3%) in acutely ill medical patients.

Hull RD, Schellong SM, Tapson VF, Monreal M, Samama MM, Nicol P, Vicaut E, Turpie AG, Yusen RD; EXCLAIM (Extended Prophylaxis for Venous Thrombo Embolism in Acutely Ill Medical Patients With Prolonged Immobilization) study. Extended-duration venous thromboembolism prophylaxis in acutely ill medical patients with recently reduced mobility: A randomized trial. *Ann Intern Med.* 2010;153(1):8–18. doi: 10.7326/0003-4819-153-1-201007060-00004. PMID: 20621900

EXCLUSION CRITERIA

Following are the exclusion criteria for the use of anticoagulation prophylaxis: bleeding disorder, abnormal clotting time, risk of bleeding, uncontrolled hypertension, hypersensitivity to UFH/LMWH, severe renal failure, **pregnancy** and intracranial/intraocular surgery where even a small risk of bleeding can be dangerous.

EXERCISE

Static exercises of the quadriceps, calf and the toes should be started as soon as possible on the day of surgery.

EXPENSES

VTE-related healthcare expenses are estimated to be about $1.5 billion every year in the United States.

EXPERT STUDY

No hematoma was reported in 1,553 patients undergoing major orthopaedic surgery with indwelling **epidural** catheter – **fondaparinux** was withheld for 48 hours before the removal of the catheter.

E

Singelyn FJ, Verheyen CC, Piovella F, Van Aken HK, Rosencher N; EXPERT Study Investigators. The safety and efficacy of extended thromboprophylaxis with fondaparinux after major orthopedic surgery of the lower limb with or without a neuraxial or deep peripheral nerve catheter: The EXPERT Study. *Anesth Analg.* 2007;105(6):1540–47. doi:10.1213/01.ane.0000287677.95626.60

EXTENDED PROPHYLAXIS
Extended prophylaxis for up to 4–5 weeks after operation is indicated in patients who have undergone major **orthopaedic surgery** e.g. hip replacement, **hip fracture** and those who have undergone major surgery for **cancer**, **stroke** with **thrombophilia** and previous history of VTE. This may be done with **warfarin** or direct oral anticoagulants (**DOACs**).

EXTENT
The extent of the thrombus in the veins does not correlate with the symptoms and signs of DVT.

EXTRACORPOREAL CIRCULATION
Pharmacological prophylaxis is used for prevention of thrombus formation in the extracorporeal circulation during **ECMO**, **haemodialysis** or **hemofiltration**.

EXTREMITY
DVT occurs more frequently in the lower extremity than in the upper extremity.

F

FACTOR II (PROTHROMBIN)

Factor II (**prothrombin**) is converted to factor IIa (**thrombin**) by factor Xa. Thrombin then converts **fibrinogen** to **fibrin** which then forms the thrombus.

See **Coagulation cascade** also.

FACTOR V LEIDEN

Factor V Leiden is a mutated form of factor V. It is the most common cause of **inherited thrombophilia**. It increases the risk of venous thromboembolism (VTE) as much as 50–100 times.

FACTOR Xa

Factor X (in its activated form i.e. Xa) plays an important role in the **coagulation cascade** by converting **prothrombin** (factor II) to **thrombin** (factor IIa). **Fondaparinux** is a factor Xa inhibitor with once-daily (OD) dosing.

FAMILY HISTORY

A family history of deep vein thrombosis/pulmonary embolism (DVT/PE) increases the risk of VTE – it carries 3 points in the **Caprini** score.

FASCIOTOMY

Fasciotomy may rarely be required to relieve the compartment syndrome in **phlegmasia cerulea dolens**.

FATAL

Massive PE can be fatal – patients at highest risk of VTE have a 0.2–5.0% risk of fatal VTE.

FAT EMBOLISM

The clinical picture of fat embolism, commonly seen in patients with long bone fractures, may resemble that of PE.

FCD (FOOT COMPRESSION DEVICE)

See **VFP (Venous foot pump)**.

FEAR

VTE prophylaxis is highly **underutilized**. Fear of bleeding is one of the major causes of underutilization of pharmacological thromboprophylaxis. Out of 488 patients admitted in the intensive care unit (ICU) at the Jaslok Hospital, Mumbai India, thromboprophylaxis was indicated in as many as 466 (98%), but only 229 (47%)

F

received thromboprophylaxis. The most common reason cited for not using thromboprophylaxis was the fear of bleeding. This fear, however, is unfounded because the risk of major bleeding is very low with optimal use of thromboprophylaxis.

Ansari K, Dalal K, Patel M. Risk stratification and utilisation of thromboembolism prophylaxis in a medical-surgical ICU: A hospital-based study. *J Indian Med Assoc.* 2007;105(9):536, 538, 540 passim.

FEMORAL

The femoral vein is commonly used for various diagnostic and therapeutic vascular interventions. An injury can occur to the femoral vein during the attempted arterial puncture. This can cause thrombosis (Fig. F1) and subsequent narrowing of the femoral vein.

FFP (FRESH FROZEN PLASMA)

Fresh frozen plasma (FFP) along with **vitamin K** is useful to control bleeding in a patient on **warfarin.**

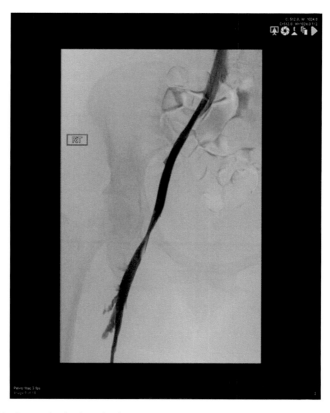

Fig. F1   Femoral vein thrombosis.

FIBRINOGEN
I^{125} tagged fibrinogen is used for **isotope venography** for the diagnosis of VTE.

FIBRINOLYSIS
Fibrinolysis with a tissue plasminogen activator (**tPA**) e.g. **streptokinase** or **urokinase** is indicated only in limb-threatening DVT and life-threatening PE.

FILARIASIS
Lymphatic filariasis, commonly known as elephantiasis, (caused by the nematode *Wuchereria bancrofti*) results in (usually) painless, firm and nonpitting oedema (lymphoedema) (Fig. F2) of the foot and leg.

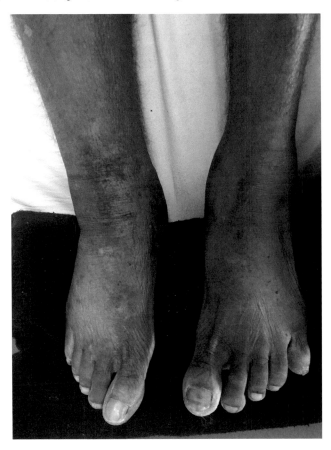

Fig. F2   Unilateral (right) nonpitting fibrosclerotic oedema (lymphedema) caused by filariasis.

FILTER

An inferior vena cava (**IVC**) filter (Fig. F3) is used to prevent PE in a select group of patients with proximal DVT in whom therapeutic anticoagulation is absolutely contraindicated e.g. recent surgery, active bleeding, haemorrhagic **stroke**; or is associated with complications or has failed; or in patients with **recurrent VTE** despite adequate anticoagulation. Prophylactic insertion of an IVC filter may be indicated in patients at a very high risk of developing PE and with contraindications to the use of thromboprophylaxis. The IVC filter is placed percutaneously through the femoral or the internal jugular (usually right) vein under fluoroscopic guidance. Earlier filters were permanent, but retrievable IVC filters are now available. IVC filters on their own are, however, associated with increased risk of recurrent DVT.

The PREPIC trial randomized 400 patients with proximal DVT to receive or not receive an IVC filter along with anticoagulation and found that the IVC filter reduced the risk of PE but increased the risk of DVT and had no effect on survival. The trial concluded that the use of IVC filters may be beneficial in patients at high risk of PE, but systematic use in the general population with VTE was not recommended.

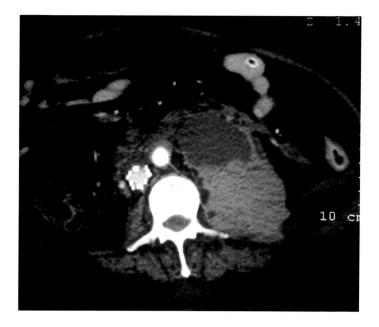

Fig. F3   Inferior vena cava (IVC) filter in situ (seen on CT) in a patient with recurrent VTE. The patient was on long-term oral anticoagulation with warfarin and also had a large hematoma (hyperdense) with liquefaction (hypodense) in the left psoas muscle.

The American College of Chest Physicians (**ACCP**), however, recommends against the use of IVC filters for thromboprophylaxis.

See **Serena Williams** also.

PREPIC Study Group. Eight-year follow-up of patients with permanent vena cava filters in the prevention of pulmonary embolism: The PREPIC (Prevention duRisque d'Embolie Pulmonaire par Interruption Cave) randomized study. *Circulation.* 2005;112(3):416–22. doi:10.1161/CIRCULATIONAHA.104.512834

FIT (FOOT IMPULSE TECHNOLOGY)

Foot impulse technology (FIT) using an **A-V impulse** system is a compression device used to promote venous flow in the foot and is one of the mechanical methods of DVT prophylaxis. It mimics the natural hemodynamic process of walking by flattening the plantar plexus and evacuating blood from the bottom of the foot.

See **VFP (venous foot pump)** also.

FLAVONOIDS, VASOACTIVE

Vasoactive flavonoids e.g. diosmin are useful in the management of **varicose veins** and haemorrhoids and NOT for VTE.

FLOW

Low-flow states e.g. prolonged immobilization, hospitalization and **long-distance** air travel promote venous thrombosis.

FLUSHING

A common problem with intravenous (IV) lines and canulae is them getting blocked with a clot. Unfractionated heparin (UFH) 10–100 IU/mL may be used to flush IV lines and canulae to prevent them getting blocked with a clot.

FONDAPARINUX

Fondaparinux is a chemical synthetic (cf. heparins which are of animal origin i.e. **porcine**-sourced) **pentasaccharide** with a molecular weight of 1,728 Da. It is a selective indirect (i.e. acting through its activation of **antithrombin**) factor **Xa** inhibitor and does not have **anti-IIa** activity. It also does not bind to platelets and, therefore, does not cause heparin-induced thrombocytopenia (**HIT**) (cf. UFH, LMWH). Fondaparinux is effective for VTE prophylaxis after **hip** and **knee replacement surgery**. It has a long half-life of 15–20 hours and can, therefore, be administered once daily (OD). Prophylactic dose is 2.5 mg SC OD starting not before 6–8 hours after surgery. This timing is possible because of the rapid onset of action of fondaparinux. Dose for treatment is 5 mg (<50 kg), 7.5 mg (50–100 kg) or 10 mg (>100 kg) SC OD (Turpie. *Arch Intern Med* 2002).

In a meta-analysis of four multicentre randomized trials including 7,344 patients undergoing major orthopaedic surgery, fondaparinux was associated with lower incidence of VTE (DVT and PE) than **enoxaparin** (6.8% vs. 13.7%).

F

Fondaparinux should be used with caution in patients who weigh <50 kg and in patients with severe **renal dysfunction** (creatinine clearance [**CC**] <30 mL/minute) and those who would require continuous **epidural** analgesia. There is no **antidote** for fondaparinux overdose; **protamine** (the antidote for heparin) is of no use.

Turpie AG, Bauer KA, Eriksson BI, Lassen MR. Fondaparinux vs enoxaparin for the prevention of venous thromboembolism in major orthopedic surgery: A meta-analysis of 4 randomized double-blind studies. *Arch Intern Med.* 2002;162(16):1833–40. doi: 10.1001/archinte.162.16.1833

FOOD INTERACTIONS

Oral anticoagulants, especially warfarin, have a lot of **interactions** with food e.g. green leafy vegetables, cauliflower, cabbage, green peas, legumes, soya bean, tomato, ginger, garlic, mango, papaya, liver, etc.; these foods should be avoided or taken in moderation.
See **Drug interactions** also.

FRACTURE

Isolated limb fracture in the absence of other risk factors does not require VTE prophylaxis. Patients with **hip fracture** and **pelvic fracture**, however, are at high risk for VTE.

FREE-FLOATING THROMBUS

The proximal end of a venous thrombus is free-floating and can break off easily to cause an embolism.

FREQUENCY OF ADMINISTRATION

UFH	3–4 times a day
LMWH	bemiparin, dalteparin, tinzaparin once daily (OD)
	enoxaparin, nadroparin twice daily (BID)

FREQUENCY OF DVT

DVT is very common in patients who do not receive VTE prophylaxis: **stroke** (55%), hip and knee replacement (50%), polytrauma (50%), **hip fracture** (45%), spinal cord injury (**SCI**) (35%), general, **gynaecological** and **neurosurgery** (25%) and myocardial infarction (**MI**) (20%).

FUT (FIBRINOGEN UPTAKE TEST)

Isotope (I^{125}) labelled **fibrinogen** is taken up by an evolving thrombus. FUT lacks the sensitivity and specificity to detect DVT. It also carries a risk of viral transmission. It is, therefore, no longer used.

G

GCS (GRADUATED COMPRESSION STOCKINGS)

Graduated compression stockings (GCS) (Fig. G1) apply a gradually decreasing pressure from the ankle through the calf and the knee to the thigh; they increase venous velocity and thus help the venous return. GCS are available as knee length or thigh length (with or without a waist belt attachment) and in variable size to fit the leg/thigh **circumference**. Choice of appropriate size and proper application (without the upper end rolling down) are important. Stockings should be worn continuously during the period of immobility.

Important measurements required to choose the correct stockings are limb and leg length and thigh and calf circumference. Inappropriate use of GCS can cause compartment syndrome, common peroneal nerve palsy and skin ulceration. Too tight stockings at the thigh level may, in fact, cause a tourniquet effect (Fig. G2) and impede venous flow, thus promoting DVT.

In a pooled analysis of randomized controlled trials (GCS $n = 624$, placebo $n = 581$), GCS alone reduced the rate of DVT from 27% to 13% (Amaragiri. *Cochrane* 2000); when combined with, low-dose unfractionated heparin (UFH), GCS reduced DVT rates from 15% to 2%.

However, recent studies suggest no additional benefit in the reduction of VTE when GCS are used along with pharmacological prophylaxis.

The presence of peripheral arterial disease causing severe or critical limb ischemia is a contraindication for the use of GCS.

Long-term use of high-pressure (>20 mm Hg) GCS was earlier advised to reduce the incidence of post-thrombotic syndrome (**PTS**) after an attack of deep vein thrombosis (DVT), but it seems that GCS do not reduce the risk of PTS after an episode of DVT.

Amaragiri SV, Lees TA. Elastic compression stockings for prevention of deep vein thrombosis. *Cochrane Database Syst Rev.* 2000;(3):CD001484. doi: 10.1002/14651858.CD001484

GECS (GRADUATED ELASTIC COMPRESSION STOCKINGS)

Graduated elastic compression stockings (GECS) is another name for graduated compression stockings (**GCS**).

GENDER

Venous thromboembolism (VTE) is slightly more common in men than in women except women of childbearing age.

See **Pregnancy**, **Puerperium** also.

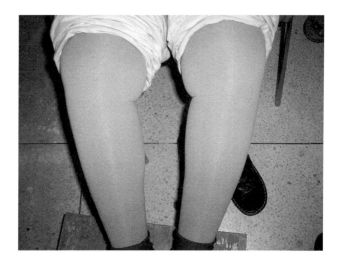

Fig. G1   Graduated compression stockings (GCS) are one of the mechanical methods of VTE prophylaxis.

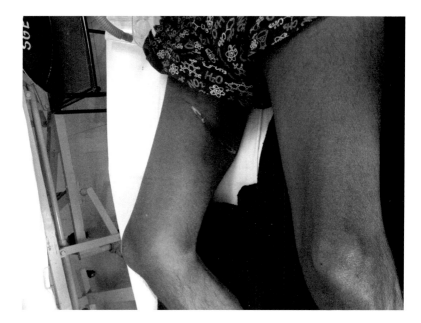

Fig. G2   Inappropriate choice and use of graduated compression stockings (GCS) can be harmful – the scar of a traumatic ulcer in the right thigh caused by a tight upper end of GCS.

GENEVA SCORE

The Geneva score (Table G1) for determining the pretest probability (**PTP**) of pulmonary embolism (PE) is calculated by adding points given to eight clinical factors: age >65 (1), previous DVT/PE (3), surgery or fracture within 1 month (2), active **cancer** (2), haemoptysis (2), unilateral lower limb pain (3), heart rate 75–94 per minute (3), pain on lower limb deep palpation and unilateral oedema (4) and heart rate (HR) ≥95 per minute (5).

A simplified Geneva score (Wicki. *Arch Intern Med* 2001) has been recently published.

Table G1   Geneva score

Geneva score	Risk of PE	Probability of PE
0–3	Low	8%
4–10	Intermediate	29%
>10	High	74%

Wicki J, Perneger TV, Junod AF, Bounameaux H, Perrier A. Assessing clinical probability of pulmonary embolism in the emergency ward: A simple score. *Arch Intern Med.* 2001;161(1):92–97. doi:10.1001/archinte.161.1.92

GOAL

The main goals of treatment of DVT are prevention of PE, recurrent DVT and post-thrombotic syndrome (**PTS**).

GREENFIELD

See **Filter, IVC filter**.

GROUP PROPHYLAXIS

There are several **strategies** for the use of VTE prophylaxis. Group prophylaxis is one of the strategies of thromboprophylaxis wherein all patients in a group of disease/procedure e.g. **cancer**, joint replacement surgery, major urological surgery receive prophylaxis. It is less cumbersome than the strategy of individual **screening**. The strategy of group prophylaxis is supported by the American College of Chest Physicians (**ACCP**). The major disadvantage of this approach is that a rare patient in the group who may not otherwise require prophylaxis also receives it. In addition, some patients in the low-risk disease/procedure group may be at high risk due to the presence of additional risk factors but may not receive prophylaxis.

GUIDELINES

G

AAFP (American Academy of Family Physicians)
https://www.aafp.org/afp/2017/0301/p295.html

AAOS (American Association of Orthopaedic Surgeons)
https://www.aaos.org/quality/quality-programs/tumor-infection-and-military-medi-cine-programs/venous-thromboembolic-disease-in-elective-tka-and-tha-prevention/

ACCP (American College of Chest Physicians)
Evidence-Based Clinical Practice Guidelines

Bates SM, Jaeschke R, Stevens SM, Goodacre S, Wells PS, Stevenson MD, Kearon C, Schunemann HJ, Crowther M, Pauker SG, Makdissi R, Guyatt GH. Diagnosis of DVT: Antithrombotic Therapy and Prevention of Thrombosis, 9th ed: American College of Chest Physicians Evidence-Based Clinical Practice Guidelines. *Chest*. 2012;141(Suppl 2):e351S–e418S. doi: 10.1378/chest.11-2299. PMID:22315267

Gould MK, Garcia DA, Wren SM, Karanicolas PJ, Arcelus JI, Heit JA, Samama CM. Prevention of VTE in nonorthopedic surgical patients: Antithrombotic Therapy and Prevention of Thrombosis, 9th ed: American College of Chest Physicians Evidence-Based Clinical Practice Guidelines. *Chest*. 2012;141(Suppl 2):e227S–77S. doi: 10.1378/chest.11-2297. PMID: 22315263

Kahn SR, Lim W, Dunn AS, Cushman M, Dentali F, Akl EA, Cook DJ, Balekian AA, Klein RC, Le H, Schulman S, Murad MH. Prevention of VTE in nonsurgical patients: Antithrombotic Therapy and Prevention of Thrombosis, 9th ed: American College of Chest Physicians Evidence-Based Clinical Practice Guidelines. *Chest*. 2012;141(Suppl 2):e195S–e226S. doi: 10.1378/chest.11-2296. PMID:22315261

Kearon C, Akl EA, Comerota AJ, Prandoni P, Bounameaux H, Goldhaber SZ, Nelson ME, Wells PS, Gould MK, Dentali F, Crowther M, Kahn SR. Antithrombotic therapy for VTE disease: Antithrombotic Therapy and Prevention of Thrombosis, 9th ed: American College of Chest Physicians Evidence-Based Clinical Practice Guidelines. *Chest*. 2012;141(Suppl 2):e419S–96S. doi: 10.1378/chest.11-2301. Erratum in: Chest. 2012 Dec;142(6):1698-1704. PMID:22315268

API (Association of Physicians of India)
http://apiindia.org/wp-content/uploads/pdf/medicine_update_2010/cardiology_31.pdf

ASCO (American Society of Clinical Oncology)
https://www.asco.org/research-guidelines/quality-guidelines/guidelines/supportive-care-and-treatment-related-issues%20#/9911

Key NS, Bohlke K, Falanga A. Venous thromboembolism prophylaxis and treatment in patients with cancer: ASCO clinical practice guideline update summary. *J Oncol Pract*. 2019;15(12):661–64. doi: 10.1200/JOP.19.00368. Epub 2019 Sep 24. No abstract available. PMID:31550210

G

Key NS, Khorana AA, Kuderer NM, Bohlke K, Lee AYY, Arcelus JI, Wong SL, Balaban EP, Flowers CR, Francis CW, Gates LE, Kakkar AK, Levine MN, Liebman HA, Tempero MA, Lyman GH, Falanga A. Venous thromboembolism prophylaxis and treatment in patients with cancer: ASCO clinical practice guideline update. *J Clin Oncol.* 2020;38(5):496–520. doi: 10.1200/JCO.19.01461. Epub 2019 Aug 5. PMID:31381464

ASH (American Society of Hematology)

Lim W, Le Gal G, Bates SM, Righini M, Haramati LB, Lang E, Kline JA, Chasteen S, Snyder M, Patel P, Bhatt M, Patel P, Braun C, Begum H, Wiercioch W, Schünemann HJ, Mustafa RA. American Society of Hematology 2018 guidelines for management of venous thromboembolism: Diagnosis of venous thromboembolism. *Blood Adv.* 2018;2(22):3226–56. doi: 10.1182/bloodadvances.2018024828. PMID:30482764

ASRA (American Society of Regional Anesthesia)

Horlocker T, Vandermeuelen E, Kopp SL; Gogarten W., Leffert LR, Benzon HT. Regional anesthesia in the patient receiving antithrombotic or thrombolytic therapy: American Society of Regional Anesthesia and Pain Medicine Evidence-Based Guidelines (Fourth Edition). *Reg Anesth Pain Med.* 2018;43(3):263–309. doi: 10.1097/AAP.0000000000000763

Australian Commission on Safety and Quality in Health Care

https://www.safetyandquality.gov.au/our-work/clinical-care-standards/venous-thromboembolism-prevention-clinical-care-standard

EAU (European Association of Urology)

https://uroweb.org/guideline/thromboprophylaxis/

European Society of Cardiology

https://www.revespcardiol.org/en-vol-68-num-1-sumario-S1885585714X00137

ESMO (European Society of Medical Oncology)

https://www.esmo.org/guidelines/supportive-and-palliative-care/venous-thromboembolism-vte-in-cancer-patients

ITAC (International Initiative on Thrombosis and Cancer)

https://www.itaccme.com/en

IUA (International Union of Angiology)

Cardiovascular Disease Educational and Research Trust; Cyprus Cardiovascular Disease Educational and Research Trust; European Venous Forum; International Surgical Thrombosis Forum; International Union of Angiology; Union Internationale de Phlébologie. Prevention and treatment of venous thromboembolism. International Consensus Statement (guidelines according to scientific evidence). *Int Angiol.* 2006;25(2):101–61. PMID: 16763532.

NCCN (National Comprehensive Cancer Network)
https://www.nccn.org/

NICE (National Institute for Health and Care Excellence)
https://www.nice.org.uk/guidance/ng89

RCOG (Royal College of Obstetricians and Gynaecologists)
https://www.rcog.org.uk/globalassets/documents/guidelines/gtg-37a.pdf

SAGES (Society of American Gastrointestinal and Endoscopic Surgeons)
VTE prophylaxis for laparoscopic surgery guidelines
https://www.sages.org/publications/guidelines/guidelines-for-deep-venous-thrombosis-prophylaxis-during-laparoscopic-surgery/

SIGN (Scottish Intercollegiate Guidelines Network)
Prophylaxis of venous thromboembolism 2002
https://www.sign.ac.uk/media/1060/sign122.pdf

In spite of the availability of several guidelines, however, VTE prophylaxis, unfortunately, remains underused.

GYNAECOLOGICAL

Patients undergoing major gynaecological surgery, especially for **cancer**, should receive prophylaxis with low-dose UFH twice or thrice daily (BID or TID) or low-molecular-weight heparin (LMWH) once daily (OD).

HAEMODIALYSIS

Heparin is used to prevent clotting in the **extracorporeal circuit** during haemodialysis.

See **Dialysis** also.

HALF-LIFE

Bemiparin, with a low molecular weight of 3,600 Da, has the longest half-life of 5.3 hours, followed by **enoxaparin** (4–5 hours), **nadroparin** (2.5 hours), **dalteparin** (2.0 hours) and **tinzaparin** (2.0 hours).

HEAD INJURY

Patients with a head injury should NOT receive **pharmacological** prophylaxis immediately after the injury – **mechanical** methods should be used instead. Pharmacological prophylaxis should be started when the risk of intracranial haemorrhage stops.

HEALTHCARE

Venous thromboembolism (VTE) is a major healthcare problem the world over, as it causes significant morbidity and mortality and results in high resource expenditure.

HELICAL CT

Helical computed tomography (CT) with pulmonary angiography (**CTPA**) is replacing conventional (invasive) **angiography** for the diagnosis of pulmonary embolism (PE).

HEMATOMA

Hematoma at the injection site is not uncommon with the use of thromboprophylaxis. This is more common with unfractionated heparin (UFH) than with low-molecular-weight heparin (LMWH). Appropriate injection technique can reduce the incidence of subcutaneous hematomas.

A hematoma can form spontaneously in the subcutaneous tissues or in the muscles (Fig. H1) following minor unnoticed trauma in patients on anticoagulants; most of these hematomas will resolve on their own. A large hematoma may liquefy and get infected to form an abscess; prophylactic antibiotics may be administered in the presence of a large hematoma.

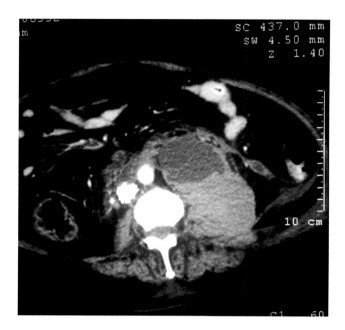

Fig. H1   A large hematoma (hyperdense) with liquefaction (hypodense) in the left psoas muscle in a patient with recurrent VTE on long-term oral anticoagulation with warfarin. Inferior vena cava (IVC) filter is also seen in situ.

HEMIPLEGIA

Patients with hemiplegia due to **stroke** have a high risk of VTE.

HEMOFILTRATION

Heparin is used to prevent clotting in the **extracorporeal circuit** during hemofiltration.

HEPARIN

The term heparin should be used to include both **UFH** and **LMWH**. Heparins have both **anti-Xa** and **anti-IIa (antithrombin)** actions.

   ANECDOTE Heparin (so named because it was isolated from the liver) was discovered in 1916 by Jay McLean (1890–1957), a second-year medical student working with Professor William H. Howell at the Johns Hopkins Medical School in Baltimore, Maryland, USA.

HEPARINOID

Heparin derivatives e.g. **danaparoid** can be used in patients with heparin-induced thrombocytopenia (**HIT**).

HEPATIC IMPAIRMENT

Patients with liver dysfunction may have deficiency of coagulation factors and have an increased risk of bleeding with thromboprophylaxis.

HEREDITARY

Patients with hereditary risk factors for VTE e.g. **factor V Leiden** mutation, prothrombin gene mutation, proteins **C** and **S** deficiency, **antithrombin** deficiency, dysfibrinogenemia and elevated levels of factor VIII may require long-term (even lifelong) thromboprophylaxis.

HFS (HIP FRACTURE SURGERY)

Patients undergoing surgery for **hip fracture** are at a very high risk for VTE. In patients with hip fracture awaiting surgery, VTE prophylaxis should begin soon after the fracture, even before the operation. Patients undergoing HFS should receive prophylaxis with LMWH or **fondaparinux**, or vitamin K antagonists (**VKA**), or low-dose unfractionated heparin (**UFH**). Fatal PE may occur in 4–13% of patients undergoing HFS without thromboprophylaxis.

HIGH RISK

The following groups of patients are at a high risk for a VTE:

- Elderly (>60 years) patients undergoing major general, **gynaecological** or urological surgery, or middle-aged (40–60 years) patients with a risk factor e.g. **cancer**
- Major trauma
- Major orthopaedic (e.g. hip **arthroplasty**, knee arthroplasty), pelvic or urological surgery; spinal cord injury (**SCI**); fracture of the pelvis, hip or lower Thrombophilia limb; **hemiplegia** or **paraplegia**

Thrombophilia

Past history of VTE (risk of VTE is as high as 40–80%)

Patients at high risk for VTE should receive higher prophylactic dose e.g. UFH thrice daily (TID) or LMWH (**bemiparin** 3,500 IU, **dalteparin** 5,000 IU, **enoxaparin** 40 mg, **nadroparin** 3,800 IU, **parnaparin** 4,250 IU) of thromboprophylaxis. Graduated compression stockings (**GCS**) and an intermittent pneumatic compression (**IPC**) device may be used in addition to pharmacological prophylaxis.

HIGHEST RISK

Patients with the highest risk of VTE are those with major trauma, spinal cord injury (**SCI**), hip **arthroplasty**, knee arthroplasty, hip fracture surgery (**HFS**) and major surgery in patients with multiple risk factors (e.g. old age, **cancer**). Incidence of VTE in this group of patients may be very high: calf deep vein thrombosis (DVT), 40–80%; proximal DVT, 10–20%; clinical PE, 4–10%; and fatal PE, 0.2–5%. These patients should receive thromboprophylaxis with both **mechanical** and **pharmacological** (higher dose) methods. These patients may require **extended prophylaxis** even after discharge from the hospital.

HIP FRACTURE
Patients with hip fracture are at a high risk for VTE.

HIP REPLACEMENT
The majority of deaths following total hip replacement (**THR**) (**arthroplasty**) are coagulation-related (i.e. because of VTE) due to inadequate thromboprophylaxis. Hip replacement surgery is one of the indications for extended (4–5 weeks) prophylaxis even after the patient is discharged from the hospital.

HIRUDINS
Hirudins e.g. **lepirudin** and desirudin are thrombin inhibitors. Lepirudin has been used in patients with heparin-induced thrombocytopenia (**HIT**).

HIT (HEPARIN-INDUCED THROMBOCYTOPENIA)
HIT occurs in about 3% of patients on UFH. A baseline platelet count should be obtained before starting any heparin whether UFH or LMWH. HIT is an immune-mediated phenomenon which usually occurs 5–10 days after starting heparin. It primarily occurs in patients on UFH but can occur with LMWH also, but the incidence is less – 2–3% with UFH and 1% with LMWH. **Fondaparinux** does not cause HIT. Heparin should be discontinued if the platelet count falls below 100,000/mm^3 or 50% of the baseline count and replaced with other agents which are less likely to cause thrombocytopenia. **Warfarin** may also be used in such patients. **Hirudins** and **danaparoid** can also be used.

HITTS (HEPARIN-INDUCED THROMBOCYTOPENIA AND THROMBOSIS SYNDROME)
Heparin-induced thrombocytopenia and thrombosis syndrome (HITTS) includes both arterial and venous thrombosis.

HISTORY OF VTE
Patients with a previous history of VTE have a very high risk of developing **recurrent** VTE, especially after hospitalization for a medical illness or after an operation.

HOME-BASED

DVT with no PE can be managed by home-based LMWH treatment. This is one of the many advantages of LMWH over UFH.

HOSPITALIZED

A large number of patients admitted to a hospital have a risk of developing VTE. Virtually all such patients have at least one risk factor, and about 40% have three or more risk factors.

However, VTE can occur in nonhospitalized patients also.

Anderson FA Jr, Spencer FA. Risk factors for venous thromboembolism. *Circulation*. 2003;107(23 Suppl 1):I9–16. doi: 10.1161/01.CIR.0000078469.07362.E6

HRT (HORMONE REPLACEMENT THERAPY)

Hormone replacement therapy (HRT) increases the risk of VTE. Patients scheduled for elective surgery should be advised to stop HRT for 4–6 weeks before surgery.

HYDRATION

Dehydration increases the risk of DVT. Adequate hydration helps to reduce the risk of DVT.

HYPERCOAGULABILITY

Age, **inherited** risk factors, active **cancer**, **oestrogen** therapy, **pregnancy** and **puerperium** act as risk factors for VTE due to hypercoagulability. Hypercoagulability following major orthopaedic surgery e.g. hip and knee replacement continues even after discharge from the hospital – it may be 3 months for hip and 4 weeks for knee replacement. This justifies **extended** VTE prophylaxis in these cases.

HYPERSENSITIVITY

Hypersensitivity to heparin or **porcine** products is a contraindication for the use of heparins. This can manifest as anaphylaxis, urticaria and angio-oedema.

IBD (INFLAMMATORY BOWEL DISEASE)
Inflammatory bowel disease (IBD), e.g. Crohn's disease and ulcerative colitis, is a risk factor for VTE.

ICU (INTENSIVE CARE UNIT)
Most patients admitted to the intensive care unit (ICU) have a high risk of VTE and are candidates for VTE prophylaxis. A common misconception or myth is that VTE occurs only in critically ill patients admitted in the ICU. While it is true that such patients are at very high risk of developing venous thromboembolism (VTE), it is very important to remember that VTE can and does occur in non-critically ill patients admitted in the general (non-ICU) wards also.

In a study of 5,451 patients with deep vein thrombosis/pulmonary embolism (DVT/PE) (diagnosed on ultrasound [US]) half were hospitalized – as many as 78% of those who were hospitalized were not admitted in the ICU.

In another study, US **screening** revealed DVT to be present in as many as 33% of medical patients admitted in the ICU.

Goldhaber SZ, Tapson VF; DVT FREE Steering Committee. A prospective registry of 5,451 patients with ultrasound-confirmed deep vein thrombosis. *Am J Cardiol.* 2004;93(2):259–62. doi: 10.1016/j.amjcard.2003.09.057

IDARUCIZUMAB
Idarucizumab is a monoclonal antibody (MCA) which quickly reverses the anticoagulant activity of dabigatran.

IDIOPATHIC DVT
Patients with idiopathic DVT should be screened for an occult **cancer**, as about 10% of patients with idiopathic VTE may have an **occult** cancer. The cancer may not be immediately detectable and may show up during the follow-up in the next 1–2 years.

IDIOPATHIC PAH (PULMONARY ARTERIAL HYPERTENSION)
Anticoagulants, along with diuretics and digoxin, are used for the treatment of idiopathic pulmonary arterial hypertension (**PAH**).

IDRAPARINUX
Idraparinux is a factor Xa inhibitor – it has a long half-life and the advantage of once-a-week administration.

A systematic review, however, found that there is not sufficient evidence to show that idraparinux and idrabiotaparinux are as effective and safe as the standard warfarin treatment for VTE prevention. Hence, Sanofi has discontinued its development.

ILIOFEMORAL VEIN THROMBOSIS
It is the condition where proximal veins such as the common iliac, external iliac and femoral veins are involved in DVT.

IMMOBILIZATION
Prolonged immobilization is a risk factor for DVT. Patients should be encouraged and helped to mobilize as soon as possible.

IMPEDANCE PLETHYSMOGRAPHY
Impedance plethysmography (IPG) records electrical impedance in the calf following temporary compression occlusion of the proximal veins by applying a cuff in the thigh. IPG, however, is not a sensitive or specific investigation for the diagnosis of DVT and is no longer used in clinical practice.

IMPLEMENTATION
For proper implementation of VTE prophylaxis, it is recommended to include it in the clinical pathways, staff manuals, departmental guidelines, hospital newsletters, etc.

IMPROVE
Multinational (Asia, Canada and Europe) observational study of 15,156 acutely ill medical patients – as many as 59% of the patients did not receive any prophylaxis and only 60% of those at risk received some prophylaxis.

Tapson VF, Decousus H, Pini M, et al. Venous thromboembolism prophylaxis in acutely ill hospitalized medical patients: Findings from the International Medical Prevention Registry on Venous Thromboembolism. *Chest.* 2007; 132(3):936–45. doi: 10.1378/chest.06-2993

IMPROVE BLEEDING RISK SCORE
The IMPROVE bleeding risk score estimates the risk of bleeding among acutely ill hospitalized patients. Factors e.g. **age**, gender, renal and liver function, platelet count, **ICU**/critical care unit (CCU) admission, central venous catheter (**CVC**) placement, active **peptic ulcer**, prior bleeding, rheumatic disease, active **malignancy** are given points from 1.0 to 4.5 (Table I1).

The points are added to calculate a score.

- Score ≥7: Increased risk of bleeding
- Score <7: No increased risk of bleeding

Table I1   IMPROVE bleeding risk score

Risk factor	Value	Point
Age	≥85 years	3.5
	40–84	1.5
	<40	0
Gender	Male	1.0
	Female	0
Renal function glomerular filtration rate (GFR)	<30 mL/min/m²	2.5
	30–59 mL/min/m²	1.0
	≥60 mL/min/m²	0
Liver function international normalized ratio (INR)	≥1.5	2.5
	≤1.5	0
Platelet count	<50,000	4.0
	>50,000	0
ICU or CCU		2.5
Central venous catheter		2.0
Active peptic ulcer		4.5
Prior bleeding within 3 months		4.0
Rheumatic disease		2.0
Active malignancy		2.0

INADEQUATE

Inadequate (in terms of the timing of initiation, dose or duration) use of thromboprophylaxis may not be effective; hence, it is important to start it in time and use it in an appropriate dose and for the appropriate duration.

INCIDENCE

Reported incidence of DVT varies widely due to the heterogeneity of the study populations and the methods used for the diagnosis of DVT. VTE is a major health problem – the annual incidence of DVT is about 100–150 per 100,000 per year, of symptomatic nonfatal PE is about 20 and of fatal (autopsy-detected) PE is about 50 per 100,000 per year. The highest incidence of DVT detected by **screening (symptomatic + subclinical)** without prophylaxis is seen in patients with **stroke** (55%), hip **arthroplasty** (50%), polytrauma (50%), knee arthroplasty (45%), **hip fracture** (45%), spinal cord injury (**SCI**) (35%), and major **gynaecological** surgery (20%).

Incidence of DVT in the population in the United States is 50–100 per 100,000 per year. DVT occurs in 10–20% of medical and 15–40% of surgical patients who do not receive prophylaxis. Incidence of DVT without prophylaxis in general surgery

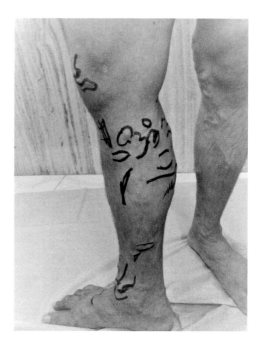

Fig. I1   Varicose veins. (Image courtesy Dr Brijesh Singh, SGPGIMS, Lucknow.)

(low to moderate risk) is 20–25% and in major orthopaedic surgery (high risk) is 40–50%. Incidence in medical patients without prophylaxis is lower i.e. 10–40%.

PE occurs in 20–25 per 100,000 hospitalized patients.

INCOMPETENCE
DVT leads to venous valvular incompetence causing **varicose veins** (Fig. I1) and venous hypertension that leads to **venous ulcer**.

INDICATION
Pharmacological prophylaxis is not indicated in low-risk patients e.g. young age, benign disease, minor surgery.

INDIVIDUAL PATIENT RISK ASSESSMENT
One of the strategies for VTE prophylaxis is to screen each patient for his or her VTE risk. This is, however, more cumbersome than **group prophylaxis**. Another easier strategy is **default prophylaxis**.

IND-PROVE (INDIAN PROSPECTIVE REGISTRY ON VTE)
Multicentre (80 centres) observational registry from May 2004 to May 2005. Studied 1,784 patients with US-diagnosed DVT. Factors causing DVT were

immobilization in 33%, previous surgery in 19% and **cancer** in 10%. Ten percent had symptoms suggestive of PE, and 8% had PE.

INFARCT
Peripheral PE may result in a pulmonary infarct. Symptoms of a pulmonary infarct include pleuritic chest pain, fever, cough and haemoptysis; examination reveals tachypnoea, tachycardia and pleural rub. **Chest X-ray** shows pleura-based opacity, but this is seen only after 5–7 days. Ventilation-perfusion (**V/Q**) scan and CT pulmonary angiography (**CTPA**) may help in diagnosis.

INFLAMMATORY BOWEL DISEASE (IBD)
Inflammatory bowel disease (IBD), e.g. Crohn's disease and ulcerative colitis is a risk factor for VTE.

INFRAPOPLITEAL DVT
DVT occurring in the veins distal to the popliteal vein; there is controversy about its treatment i.e. whether anticoagulation should be given or not.

INHERITED
Inherited risk factors for VTE e.g. protein **C** and **S** deficiency, **antithrombin** deficiency, factor V **Leiden** mutation and prothrombin mutation increase the risk of VTE almost 10-fold.

INITIATION
Initiation of low-molecular-weight (LMWH) prophylaxis before or after surgery – both are acceptable options. Surgeons in the United States prefer to start thromboprophylaxis 12–24 hours after surgery to reduce the risk of bleeding; this is in contrast to the practice of the European surgeons, who prefer to start prophylaxis 8–12 hours preoperatively. Another advantage of starting prophylaxis after surgery is that the patient can be admitted on the day of surgery; on the other hand, if prophylaxis has to start before surgery, the patient will have to be admitted the previous day. LMWH started 1 hour before surgery vs. 6 hours after surgery had a better effect but a greater risk of bleeding. Low doses of LMWH, indicated in moderate-risk patients, may be given 2 hours before surgery. High doses of LMWH, indicated in high-risk patients, should, however, be given 10–12 hours before surgery. **Fondaparinux** is started 6–8 hours after surgery has finished.

INR (INTERNATIONAL NORMALIZED RATIO)
International normalized ratio (INR) is a calculated value derived from the prothrombin time (PT) based on the international sensitivity index of the reagents used for the estimation of PT.

INR is used for the monitoring of oral anticoagulation treatment with **warfarin** – the goal is to maintain INR between 2.0 and 3.0. INR is to be done twice a week in the first week, once a week for a month and then every 2–3 weeks.

INTERACTIONS

Oral anticoagulants, especially **warfarin**, have lot of pharmacological interactions with many other **drugs** and **foods**, which should be kept in mind.

See **Drug interactions, Food interactions** also.

INTERNATIONAL UNION OF ANGIOLOGY (IUA)

See **IUA**.

INTRAMUSCULAR (IM)

Heparin should NOT be injected intramuscularly (IM); it should be administered subcutaneously (SC).

INTRAOPERATIVE

In about half of the cases with VTE, the thrombotic process starts during the operation itself – hence the importance of starting thromboprophylaxis preoperatively.

INVESTIGATIONS

Investigations useful for the diagnosis of DVT include **D-dimer**, **Doppler** US, isotope **venography**, conventional contrast venography and magnetic resonance (MR) venography; of these, contrast venography and MR venography have the highest sensitivity (almost 100%) and specificity (almost 100%). The sensitivity of most tests is higher for symptomatic (more than 90%) than for **asymptomatic** (**silent**) (50–60%) DVT. D-dimer has a very low (about 50%) specificity.

Investigations for the diagnosis of PE include electrocardiogram (**ECG**), **echo**, **V/Q** isotope lung scan, conventional pulmonary angiography, CT pulmonary angiography (**CTPA**) and MR pulmonary angiography (**MRPA**). CTPA remains the most common investigation used for the diagnosis of PE.

IPC (INTERMITTENT PNEUMATIC COMPRESSION)

To prevent DVT, the compression should be circumferential, sequential and graduated. Intermittent pneumatic compression (IPC) compresses the ankle (45 mm Hg), calf (40 mm Hg) and thigh (30 mm Hg) but not the popliteal fossa (0 mm Hg) for about 10 seconds/minute. It prevents venous stasis by causing pulsatile emptying of the veins and thus helps venous return in the lower limbs. It is a noninvasive mechanical method of thromboprophylaxis and has no risk of bleeding (cf. pharmacological methods) and should be liberally used. It must, however, be ensured that the device is properly applied. IPC may cause sweating, skin irritation, itching and an unpleasant feeling of heat and pressure. IPC in elderly diabetics with peripheral neuropathy should be used with caution, as it may cause an ulcer. IPC should not be used in presence of DVT, as it can promote

PE. IPC is also contraindicated in patients with congestive heart failure (CHF) and peripheral arterial disease (PAD).

In a pooled analysis of 11 randomized controlled trials (**RCTs**), IPC reduced the incidence of DVT from 7% to 2%. IPC is more effective than graduated compression stockings (**GCS**) in high-risk patients.

See **A-V Impulse System** also.

ITAC

The International Initiative on Thrombosis and Cancer (ITAC) is aimed at establishing a global consensus for the treatment and prophylaxis of VTE in patients with **cancer** and has developed an app for its **guidelines**.

https://www.itaccme.com/en

IUA (INTERNATIONAL UNION OF ANGIOLOGY)

Cardiovascular Disease Educational and Research Trust; Cyprus Cardiovascular Disease Educational and Research Trust; European Venous Forum; International Surgical Thrombosis Forum; International Union of Angiology; Union Internationale de Phlébologie. Prevention and treatment of venous thromboembolism. International Consensus Statement (guidelines according to scientific evidence). *Int Angiol.* 2006;25(2):101–61. PMID: 16763532.

IVC (GREENFIELD) FILTER

An inferior vena cava (IVC) filter (Fig. I2) is indicated in the presence of DVT to prevent PE, if anticoagulation therapy is contraindicated or it causes significant complications. The filter is also indicated in the presence of a fresh incidence of PE in spite of adequate anticoagulation. The IVC filter should be placed before **thrombectomy** is attempted in the presence of a free-floating thrombus. It decreases the risk of PE but may be associated with an increased risk of recurrent DVT at the insertion site. The IVC filter can be inserted at the bedside with US guidance. **Retrievable** filters are also available.

There are very few indications for IVC filter placement these days; anticoagulation remains the mainstay of treatment of DVT and prevention of PE.

See **Filter** also.

IVC (INFERIOR VENA CAVA) INTERRUPTION

IVC interruption by a **filter** to prevent PE in patients with established DVT.

IVC (INFERIOR VENA CAVA) THROMBOSIS

IVC thrombosis (Fig. I3) presents with bilateral pedal oedema.

IVUS

Intravascular ultrasound (IVUS) is sometimes used for the treatment of venous obstruction and placement of inferior vena cava (IVC) **filter**.

I

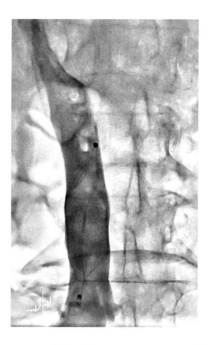

Fig. I2 Inferior vena cava (IVC) filter seen on venography. (Image courtesy Dr Saurabh Galodha, AIIMS, New Delhi.)

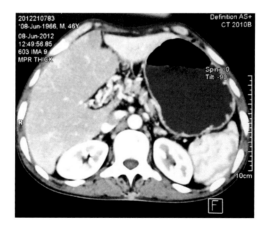

Fig. I3 Thrombus (hypodense) in the inferior vena cava (IVC).

J

JAUNDICE

Patients with surgical obstructive jaundice have coagulopathy manifesting as prolonged prothrombin time (PT) and international normalized ratio (**INR**). This is treated with **vitamin K**. The patient may, at the same time, have a pro-thrombotic state because of the disease e.g. cancer that caused the jaundice. Careful prophylaxis is, therefore, required.

K

KAKKAR, V.V.

In a landmark study published in *Lancet* in 1975, the late Prof V.V. Kakkar showed that unfractionated heparin (UFH) saved 7 lives for every 1,000 operations. A reported 4,121 patients undergoing major surgery were randomized to receive UFH (5,000 IU 2 hours before surgery and then every 8 hours for 7 days) or nothing only. Eighty patients died in the UFH group vs. 100 in the control group. The number of patients with fatal pulmonary embolism (PE) was only 2 in the UFH group (cf. 16 in the control group).

Kakkar VV. Prevention of fatal postoperative pulmonary embolism by low doses of heparin. An international multicentre trial. *Lancet*. 1975;2(7924):45–51. PMID: 49649.

KIDNEY

Low-molecular-weight heparins (LMWHs) are excreted through the kidneys. Their dose, therefore, needs to be adjusted in patients with **renal dysfunction**. This is guided by the **creatinine clearance (CC).**

KNEE REPLACEMENT

Venous thromboembolism (VTE) is common after knee replacement (**arthroplasty**). Knee replacement surgery is one of the indications for extended (4–5 weeks) prophylaxis even after the patient is discharged from the hospital.

See **Knee arthroplasty, TKR, Total knee replacement** also.

K, VITAMIN

Bleeding in a patient on **warfarin** may require blood transfusion, fresh frozen plasma (**FFP**) and vitamin K administration.

L

LAPAROSCOPIC CHOLECYSTECTOMY
Patients undergoing laparoscopic cholecystectomy in 30–45 minutes do not need venous thromboembolism (VTE) prophylaxis unless additional **risk factors** are present.

LAPAROSCOPIC SURGERY
Patients undergoing laparoscopic surgery are at a higher risk of VTE because of the anti-Trendelenburg position during the operation and venous stasis caused by the compression of the inferior vena cava (IVC) and the iliac veins due to the pneumoperitoneum. High intraperitoneal pressures should be avoided and the pneumoperitoneum released intermittently to promote venous flow.

Patients who do not have other risk factors for VTE and who are undergoing laparoscopic procedures in 30–45 minutes, however, do not need thromboprophylaxis.

LDT (LONG-DISTANCE TRAVEL)
Long-distance travel (LDT) is defined as a flight >6 hours duration. It increases the risk of deep vein thrombosis (DVT). To lessen this risk, one should avoid constrictive clothing, wear loose clothes, avoid alcohol, avoid **dehydration**, drink plenty of fluids and do frequent calf muscle stretching exercises; below-knee graduated compression stockings (**GCS**) may also be worn by those with a previous history of VTE. In the presence of factors predisposing to an increased risk of VTE, prophylaxis with a single dose of low-molecular-weight heparin (LMWH) prior to departure may be used.

LDUH
Low-dose unfractionated heparin (UFH) (LDUH) is used for VTE prophylaxis and treatment. The dose for prophylaxis is 5,000 U SC BID or TID. Prophylactic use of UFH does not require monitoring with activated partial thromboplastin time (**aPTT**). Dose for treatment is 80 U/kg intravenous (IV) bolus then IV infusion 18 U/kg 1,000–2,000 U/hour (dose is guided by aPTT every 6 hours, with the aPTT target being at least one and a half times greater than control).

LEGAL LIABILITY
A physician or surgeon who omits thromboprophylaxis in patients with the highest or high risk for VTE may be liable to a medico-legal suit by the patient because the role and usefulness of thromboprophylaxis in such patients is well-established.

LEIDEN
See **Factor V Leiden**.

LEPIRUDIN
Lepirudin is a derivative of **hirudin** – a thrombin inhibitor derived from leeches. It is useful to treat DVT in patients with heparin-induced thrombocytopenia (**HIT**). A loading intravenous (IV) dose of 0.4 mg/kg is followed by a continuous IV infusion of 0.15 mg/kg per hour.

LETHAL
Pulmonary embolism (PE) is a dangerous, even potentially lethal, complication of DVT.

LEVEL
Levels of risk (Table L1) of VTE are classified as low, moderate, high and very high.

Table L1   Levels of risk of VTE

Risk level	Frequency of VTE %		
	DVT	Proximal DVT	Fatal PE
Low	10	1	0.01
Moderate	10–40	1–10	0.1–1.0
High	40–80	10–30	1–10

LEVEL OF EVIDENCE
Also called the hierarchy of evidence

I: Systematic review or meta-analysis of all relevant randomized controlled trials (**RCTs**), or evidence-based clinical practice guidelines based on systematic reviews of RCTs, or three or more RCTs of good quality that have similar results

II: One well-designed, large, multisite RCT

III: Well-designed but nonrandomized controlled trials

IV: Well-designed case-control or cohort studies

V: Systematic reviews of descriptive and qualitative studies (meta-synthesis)

VI: Single descriptive or qualitative study

VII: Opinion of authorities and/or reports of expert committees

LIFE-THREATENING
PE is a dangerous, potentially life-threatening, complication of DVT.

LITHOTOMY

The lithotomy position during surgery e.g. urological, **gynaecological**, pelvic increases the risk of VTE.

L

LIVER DISEASE

In liver disease, prothrombin time (**PT**) and international normalized ratio (**INR**) are prolonged, but there is a higher risk of VTE because protein **C** and **S** and **antithrombin 3**, which are synthesized in the liver, are deficient. Careful anticoagulation (along with vitamin K) may be used.

LIVES

The Joint Commission on Accreditation of Healthcare Organizations (JCAHO) says that VTE prophylaxis can save lives.

LMWH (LOW-MOLECULAR-WEIGHT HEPARIN)

LMWHs are obtained by fractionation or depolymerization of polymeric heparin. They have more **anti-Xa** than **anti-IIa** activity. The anti-Xa activity of LMWH is through its activation of **antithrombin 3**, which then binds to and inhibits factor Xa. By definition, a LMWH should have a mean molecular weight <4,000 Da (cf. heparin 20,000 Da), less than 15% of the chains should have molecular weight >6,000 Da and anti-Xa to anti-IIa ratio should be >4:1 (higher than UFH 1:1). LMWHs resemble UFH in that they bind to and activate antithrombin; unlike UFH, however, they do not bind to and do not inactivate thrombin (factor IIa). Unlike UFH, LMWHs do not need **monitoring** with activated partial thromboplastin time (**aPTT**). LMWHs have a longer half-life; thus a single daily dose is needed (UFH has a shorter half-life and requires two to three doses per day). They can be administered to non-hospitalized patients also.

LMWHs have better bioavailability and a more predictable anticoagulation response than UFH. LMWHs cause less heparin-induced thrombocytopenia (**HIT**) and less **osteoporosis** than UFH. LMWHs also cause less **bleeding** and **hematoma** than UFH. LMWHs are superior to UFH, in terms of recurrence and death, for the initial treatment of DVT. They are, however, more expensive than UFH. For the treatment of PE, LMWHs are as effective and as safe as UFH.

LMWHs work best when started between 2 hours preoperatively or 6–8 hours postoperatively.

A meta-analysis of nine trials including 4,669 patients showed that the risk of major bleeding is less with LMWH than with UFH.

Protamine, which can reverse the effect of heparin, has limited effect on LMWHs. In case bleeding occurs, platelet transfusion is required.

Mismetti P, Laporte-Simitsidis S, Tardy B, Cucherat M, Buchmüller A, Juillard-Delsart D, Decousus H. Prevention of venous thromboembolism in internal

L

medicine with unfractionated or low-molecular-weight heparins: A meta-analysis of randomised clinical trials. *Thromb Haemost.* 2000;83(1):14–19. PMID: 10669147.

LONG-DISTANCE TRAVEL
See **LDT (Long-distance travel).**

LOW-DOSE UNFRACTIONATED HEPARIN (LDUH)
See **LDUH**

LOWER LIMBS
DVT of the lower limbs, especially the iliofemoral veins, is much more common and clinically important; but DVT can, rarely though, occur in the **subclavian** veins, visceral veins and the inferior vena cava (IVC).

LOWER LIMB INJURY
Patients with an isolated lower limb fracture do not need VTE prophylaxis if early mobilization can be assured and if there are no other risk factors for VTE.

LOW-MOLECULAR-WEIGHT HEPARIN (LMWH)
See **LMWH**.

LOW-RISK
Low-risk patients for VTE are those undergoing minor (less than 30–45 minutes) surgery or young (<40 years) ambulant patients, with no risk factor, minor trauma and ambulant medical patients. Patients with a low risk have a 96% chance of not having DVT; this becomes 99% if **D-dimer** is negative.

Patients at low risk of VTE do not require prophylaxis – adequate **hydration** and early **ambulation** alone are enough. Graduated compression stockings (**GCS**) and intermittent pneumatic compression (**IPC**) may be used.

LUNG ATTACK
Just as coronary artery thrombosis causes a heart attack, DVT can cause a 'lung attack' in the form of PE.

LYMPH NODE DISSECTION
Patients with pelvic (including **gynaecological**) **cancer**s who undergo pelvic lymph node dissection are at a high risk for VTE.

MAJOR

Major (lasting for >45 minutes) surgery is a risk factor for deep vein thrombosis (DVT).

MALIGNANCY

See **Cancer**.

MASSIVE

A massive PE causes hemodynamic instability in the form of hypotension/shock (systolic blood pressure <100 mm Hg); it may be fatal and can cause sudden death. It requires treatment with systemic **thrombolysis**; **thrombectomy** (surgical or **endovascular**) may be required.

MATISSE-DVT

Randomized, double-blind trial of 2,205 patients with acute symptomatic DVT. **Fondaparinux** SC once daily (OD) was as effective as **enoxaparin** 1 mg/kg SC twice daily (BID) in the treatment of symptomatic DVT. Recurrent VTE occurred in 3.9% vs. 4.1%; major bleeding in 1.1% vs. 1.2% patients.

Büller HR, Davidson BL, Decousus H, Gallus A, Gent M, Piovella F, Prins MH, Raskob G, Segers AE, Cariou R, Leeuwenkamp O, Lensing AW; Matisse Investigators. Fondaparinux or enoxaparin for the initial treatment of symptomatic deep venous thrombosis: A randomized trial. *Ann Intern Med.* 2004; 140(11):867–73. doi: 10.7326/0003-4819-140-11-200406010-00007. PMID: 15172900.

MATISSE-PE

Randomized, open-label trial of 2,213 patients with acute symptomatic PE. **Fondaparinux** SC once daily (OD) was as effective and as safe as intravenous (IV) unfractionated heparin (UFH) in the treatment of PE. Recurrent VTE occurred in 3.8% vs. 5.0%; major bleeding in 1.3% vs. 1.1% patients.

Büller HR, Davidson BL, Decousus H, Gallus A, Gent M, Piovella F, Prins MH, Raskob G, van den Berg-Segers AE, Cariou R, Leeuwenkamp O, Lensing AW; Matisse Investigators. Subcutaneous fondaparinux versus intravenous unfractionated heparin in the initial treatment of pulmonary embolism. *N Engl J Med.* 2003;349(18):1695–702. doi: 10.1056/NEJMoa035451. Erratum in: *N Engl J Med.* 2004;350(4):423. PMID: 14585937.

M

MAY THURNER SYNDROME

This is a narrowing of the left common iliac vein (Fig. M1) caused by its compression by the right common iliac artery against the spine, seen more frequently in women. It remains unrecognized until the development of DVT during **pregnancy** or until the patient develops symptoms and signs of venous hypertension. Current treatment protocol involves **thrombolytic therapy**, anticoagulation and iliac vein **stenting** as a limb salvage procedure in the acute situation, when the limb is threatened by **phlegmasia cerulea dolens** and to prevent post-thrombotic syndrome (**PTS**).

MECHANICAL METHODS

Mechanical methods for VTE prophylaxis include **ambulation**, graduated compression stockings (**GCS**), electrical calf stimulation, intermittent pneumatic compression (**IPC**) and mechanical venous foot pumps (**VFPs**).

Patients should be asked to continue ambulation at home (before the hospitalization for elective surgery), during the hospitalization and after discharge from the hospital. Proper positioning of the patient on the operation table with adequate padding to avoid pressure is important.

Mechanical methods should be used with caution in elderly patients, as their use may restrict the mobilization of these patients and may, thus, have a negative effect.

Mechanical methods are useful in patients with contraindications to the use of **pharmacological** prophylaxis. They may also be used as an adjunct to pharmacological prophylaxis. It is important to select the correct size, apply the device properly and

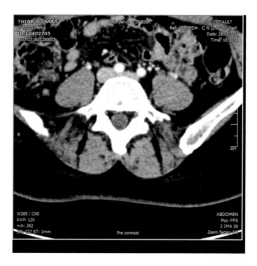

Fig. M1   May Thurner syndrome – compression of the left common iliac vein caused by the right common iliac artery.

ensure that they are worn at all times. Mechanical methods need strict compliance from the patients (cf. pharmacological prophylaxis) which is healthcare-based.

Mechanical methods, however, are less effective than pharmacological prophylaxis. Mechanical methods have the big advantage over pharmacological prophylaxis in that there is no risk of bleeding.

MEDENOX STUDY

Double-blind, placebo-controlled, randomized study to evaluate **enoxaparin** in medical patients.

Thromboprophylaxis with low-molecular-weight heparin (LMWH) (enoxaparin 20/40 mg SC daily) for 6–14 days reduced the incidence of venous thromboembolism (VTE) in 1,102 acutely ill medical patients. The incidence of VTE (by 14 days) was 5.5% in the enoxaparin (40 mg) group vs. 14.9% in the placebo group. The rate of proximal DVT was also less in the enoxaparin group vs. placebo (1.7% vs. 4.9%). Death occurred in 11%, 15% and 14% of patients in the enoxaparin 40 mg, 20 mg and placebo groups, respectively. Major bleeding occurred in 1.7% vs. 1.1% of patients.

See **ARTEMIS** also.

Samama MM, Cohen AT, Darmon JY, Desjardins L, Eldor A, Janbon C, Leizorovicz A, Nguyen H, Olsson CG, Turpie AG, Weisslinger N. A comparison of enoxaparin with placebo for the prevention of venous thromboembolism in acutely ill medical patients. Prophylaxis in Medical Patients with Enoxaparin Study Group. *N Engl J Med.* 1999;341(11):793–800. doi: 10.1056/NEJM199909093411103. PMID: 10477777.

MEDICAL (NONSURGICAL) PATIENTS

Severely restricted mobility due to acute illness e.g. **stroke**, **paraplegia**, myocardial infarction (**MI**), congestive heart failure (**CHF**), chronic obstructive lung disease (COLD) with chest infection, respiratory failure, acute renal failure (ARF), systemic infection (sepsis), etc., increases the risk of VTE in medical patients. About 1 in 20 such patients may develop VTE. All acutely ill hospitalized patients must be screened for the risk of VTE, and those at moderate, high or highest risk should receive VTE prophylaxis for at least 7 days or until the resolution of the acute medical illness.

About 50–70% of symptomatic VTE and 70–80% of fatal PEs occur in medical (nonsurgical) patients. One possible reason is that medical patients are older and sicker, while surgical patients are relatively younger and fitter.

In a study of 3,706 medical patients, **dalteparin** 5,000 IU SC daily reduced Doppler ultrasound (US)–screened proximal DVT, symptomatic VTE or sudden death from 5.0% to 2.8%; major bleeding occurred in 0.5% vs. 0.2% patients.

Leizorovicz A, Cohen AT, Turpie AG, Olsson CG, Vaitkus PT, Goldhaber SZ; PREVENT Medical Thromboprophylaxis Study Group. Randomized, placebo-controlled trial of dalteparin for the prevention of venous thromboembolism in acutely ill medical patients. *Circulation.* 2004;110(7):874–79. doi: 10.1161/01.CIR.0000138928.83266.24. Epub 2004 Aug 2. PMID: 15289368.

MEDICO-LEGAL ASPECT
See **Legal**.

MEGESTROL
Megestrol, commonly used to ameliorate cancer cachexia, increases the risk of VTE.

MELAGATRAN
Melagatran (as also **argatroban** and **dabigatran**) is a synthetic oral direct thrombin inhibitor (**DTI**). It was withdrawn because of reports of hepatotoxicity.

See **Ximelagatran** also.

MESENTERIC VEIN
Portal vein thrombosis may extend proximally into the superior mesenteric vein (SMV) causing venous congestion of the bowel to begin with and ischaemic gangrene in the later stages and into the splenic vein resulting in splenomegaly and gastric varices.

META-ANALYSIS
A meta-analysis is a quantitative study design to assess previous studies, usually randomized controlled trials (**RCTs**). It combines data from multiple studies. Meta-analysis of all RCTs produces the highest **level** i.e. Level 1 evidence.

In a meta-analysis of 46 randomized trials including patients undergoing general surgery, low-dose unfractionated heparin (LDUH) reduced DVT from 22% to 9%, PE from 2.0% to 1.3%, fatal PE from 0.8% to 0.3% and all-cause mortality from 4.2% to 3.2%, with an increase in bleeding from 3.8% to 5.9% (Collins. *NEJM* 1988).

A recent meta-analysis of nine studies involving 19,958 medical patients showed that VTE prophylaxis prevented DVT in 52%, PE in 56% and fatal PE in 62% of cases (Dentali. *Ann Intern Med* 2007).

Collins R, Scrimgeour A, Yusuf S, Peto R. Reduction in fatal pulmonary embolism and venous thrombosis by perioperative administration of subcutaneous heparin. Overview of results of randomized trials in general, orthopedic, and urologic surgery. *N Engl J Med*. 1988;318(18):1162–73. doi: 10.1056/NEJM198805053181805. PMID: 3283548.

Dentali F, Douketis JD, Gianni M, Lim W, Crowther MA. Meta-analysis: anticoagulant prophylaxis to prevent symptomatic venous thromboembolism in hospitalized medical patients. *Ann Intern Med*. 2007;146(4):278–88. doi: 10.7326/0003-4819-146-4-200702200-00007. PMID: 17310052.

MI (MYOCARDIAL INFARCTION)
Patients who have had an MI are at a higher risk for VTE.

Clinical picture of PE may mimic that of MI.

MISPERCEPTIONS

A lot of myths and misperceptions exist about VTE.

See **Some Myths/Misconceptions about Venous Thromboembolism (VTE)**, pp. xxxix–xl.

MOBILIZATION

Early (within 48 hours) and persistent mobilization alone is good enough for low-risk surgical patients (age <40 years, minor operation, no other VTE risk factor) – no mechanical or pharmacological prophylaxis is indicated in such cases. In moderate- or high-risk patients, mobilization is a useful adjunct to VTE prophylaxis - mechanical and pharmacological. Mechanical methods alone should be reserved for thromboprophylaxis in patients with high risk for bleeding.

MODERATE-RISK

Moderate-risk patients for VTE are middle-aged (40–60 years) patients undergoing major general, **gynaecological** or urological surgery or those undergoing nonmajor surgery but with other VTE risk factors, bed-ridden medical patients or those with major **trauma**; these patients have a 10–40% risk of developing VTE.

Patients who have moderate risk for VTE should receive prophylaxis with graduated compression stocking (**GCS**) or intermittent pneumatic compression (**IPC**) or LDUH 5,000 U BID or LMWH OD.

MODIFIABLE

There are several risk factors for VTE. Some risk factors of VTE e.g. **obesity**, **smoking**, activity level and exercise are modifiable.

MOLECULAR WEIGHT

UFH has a high molecular weight of 15,000 Da. LMWHs have lower molecular weights: **tinzaparin** 6,500 Da, **dalteparin** 5,700 Da, **parnaparin** 4,500 Da, **enoxaparin** 4,500 Da, **nadroparin** 4,300 Da. **Bemiparin**, a second-generation LMWH, is the lowest molecular weight (3,600 Da) heparin available. Higher-molecular-weight LMWHs e.g. **dalteparin** and **tinzaparin** are less dependent on renal clearance and do not need dose modification. They have less risk of accumulation and less risk of bleeding in patients with **renal dysfunction**.

MONITORING

Platelets (for thrombocytopenia) and serum potassium (for hypokalaemia) should be monitored in patients on UFH. Monitoring of **coagulation profile**, which is essential when UFH is used, is not required with LMWH. It may, however, be required in elderly, **obese** or **pregnant** patients and those with **renal dysfunction** receiving LMWH. The dosage of **warfarin** is monitored by prothrombin time/international normalized ratio (PT/**INR**).

MORTALITY

In-hospital case fatality of VTE is 12%. About 30% of patients with **massive** PE die suddenly before anything can be done for its diagnosis or management. Mortality of PE without diagnosis and treatment is as high as 30%; it can be reduced to 2–8% with timely diagnosis and proper treatment.

Six percent of patients with DVT and 12% of those with PE die within 1 month; at 1 year the mortality is about 30–35%.

In a study of 1,358 patients admitted to an acute care hospital, use of UFH (5,000 U BID) reduced the mortality from 10.9% to 7.8% (Halkin. *Ann Intern Med* 1982).

Halkin H, Goldberg J, Modan M, Modan B. Reduction of mortality in general medical in-patients by low-dose heparin prophylaxis. *Ann Intern Med.* 1982;96(5):561–65. doi: 10.7326/0003-4819-96-5-561. PMID: 7073148.

MRPA (MAGNETIC RESONANCE PULMONARY ANGIOGRAPHY)

Magnetic resonance pulmonary angiography (MRPA) with gadolinium enhancement is gradually replacing conventional angiography for the diagnosis of PE. If MR is not available or is contraindicated e.g. a metal implant, CT pulmonary angiography **(CTPA)** is an alternative.

MDCT (MULTIDETECTOR CT)

CT pulmonary angiography **(CTPA)** using multidetector CT (MDCT) for the diagnosis of PE can be done with a single 5- to 10-second breath-hold.

MULTISPECIALTY

VTE can affect patients in various specialties e.g. internal medicine, general surgery, gynaecology, orthopaedics, obstetrics, trauma, urology, intensive care, etc.

MUTATION

Mutation of factor V **Leiden** and **prothrombin** genes increases the risk of VTE.

MYELOPROLIFERATIVE

Patients with myeloproliferative disorders (MPDs) e.g. chronic myeloid leukaemia (CML), polycythaemia vera are at a high risk of developing VTE.

MYTH

The myth that VTE does not occur in Indian patients has been proven to be false by several recent studies and reports; VTE does occur in Indian patients also.

See **Some Myths/Misconceptions about Venous Thromboembolism (VTE)**, pp. xxxix–xl.

N

NADROPARIN

- Nadroparin is one of the low-molecular-weight heparins (LMWHs). Molecular weight is 4,300 Da, half-life is 2.5 hours and a**nti-Xa** to **anti-IIa** ratio is 3.0:1.
- Dose for prophylaxis of venous thromboembolism (VTE) is 2,850/3,800 IU SC OD.
- Dose for the treatment of VTE is 4,100 IU SC BID.

NAFT (NORTH AMERICAN FRAGMIN TRIAL)
A randomized, double-blind trial in 569 patients undergoing hip **arthroplasty** showed that a regimen of **dalteparin** (Fragmin[R] Pfizer) begun early postoperatively (mean 6 hours) was as effective as a preoperative regimen and more effective than **warfarin** for preventing deep vein thrombosis (**DVT**). Dalteparin did not increase clinically important bleeding complications as compared to warfarin.

Hull RD, Pineo GF, Francis C, Bergqvist D, Fellenius C, Soderberg K, Holmqvist A, Mant M, Dear R, Baylis B, Mah A, Brant R. Low-molecular-weight heparin prophylaxis using dalteparin extended out-of-hospital vs in-hospital warfarin/out-of-hospital placebo in hip arthroplasty patients: A double-blind, randomized comparison. North American Fragmin Trial Investigators. *Arch Intern Med.* 2000;160(14):2208–15. doi: 10.1001/archinte.160.14.2208. PMID: 10904465.

NATIONAL INSTITUTE FOR HEALTH AND CARE EXCELLENCE (NICE)
See **NICE**.

NCCN (NATIONAL COMPREHENSIVE CANCER NETWORK)
The National Comprehensive Cancer Network (NCCN) guidelines are followed by the clinicians all over the world for the management of cancer patients. NCCN recommends VTE prophylaxis for all abdominal and pelvic oncologic resections.

Streiff MB, Holmstrom B, Angelini D, Ashrani A, Bockenstedt PL, Chesney C, Fanikos J, Fenninger RB, Fogerty AE, Gao S, Goldhaber SZ, Gundabolu K, Hendrie P, Lee AI, Lee JT, Mann J, McMahon B, Millenson MM, Morton C, Ortel TL, Ozair S, Paschal R, Shattil S, Siddiqi T, Smock KJ, Soff G,

Wang TF, Williams E, Zakarija A, Hammond L, Dwyer MA, Engh AM. NCCN Guidelines Insights: Cancer-Associated Venous Thromboembolic Disease, Version 2.2018. *J Natl ComprCancNetw.* 2018;16(11):1289–1303. doi: 10.6004/jnccn.2018.0084. PMID: 30442731.

NEGLECTED
VTE prophylaxis, though important, is one of the neglected areas of healthcare.

NEPHROTIC SYNDROME
Nephrotic syndrome is a risk factor for VTE.

NEURAXIAL (EPIDURAL/SPINAL) ANAESTHESIA
The best time to place or remove a spinal or epidural needle/catheter (Fig. N1) is when the anticoagulant effect of thromboprophylaxis is at its lowest i.e. 8–12 hours after the last dose of unfractionated heparin (UFH) or 24 hours after the last dose of LMWH. LMWH can be started 6–8 hours after surgery, and the next dose should be given 24 hours after this dose. The catheter should be removed just before the next dose is due, and the next dose should be administered 2 hours after the removal of the catheter.

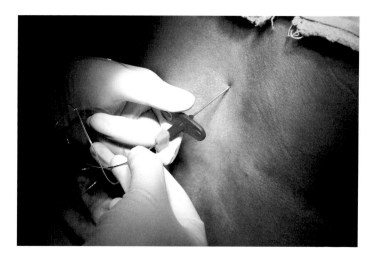

Fig. N1 Neuraxial e.g. epidural anaesthesia and analgesia are frequently used in major operations; caution needs to exercised while placing and removing the catheter in patients receiving VTE prophylaxis.

A reported 1,264 patients undergoing major orthopaedic surgery received **bemiparin** started 6 hours postoperatively; 1,116 of these patients received neuraxial anaesthesia and no spinal/epidural hematoma was observed.

Spinal hematoma is a rare complication of spinal/epidural puncture in patients on pharmacological prophylaxis. It manifests as severe low back pain and weakness of the lower limbs. Early decompression by laminectomy may be beneficial. If treatment is delayed, it may result in permanent paralysis of the lower limbs.

See **ASRA (American Society of Regional Anesthesia)** also.

NEUROSURGERY
Patients undergoing major neurosurgery e.g. craniotomy for brain tumour are at risk for VTE and should receive VTE prophylaxis with **mechanical** methods; heparins may be started postoperatively. This does not increase the risk of bleeding.

Graduated compression stockings (**GCS**) with LMWH was associated with less DVT than GCS alone, with no significant increase in the risk of intracranial bleed. LMWH is started 12 hours after surgery.

NEWER ANTICOAGULANTS
Newer oral anticoagulants (**NOA** or **NOAC**) e.g. **apixaban**, **edoxaban** and **rivaroxaban** (**anti-Xa**) and **dabigatran** (**anti-IIa**). **Ximelagatran (melagatran)** has been withdrawn from clinical use due to hepatic toxicity.

NICE (NATIONAL INSTITUTE FOR HEALTH AND CARE EXCELLENCE)
https://www.nice.org.uk/guidance/ng89

NOA OR NOAC
Novel oral anticoagulants (NOAs or NOACs) are specific inhibitors of factor Xa (activated) e.g. **apixaban**, **edoxaban**, **rivaroxaban** or of thrombin i.e. factor IIa (**dabigatran**).

Also called direct anticoagulants (**DOACs**).

NONSPECIFIC
Symptoms and signs of deep venous thrombosis (DVT) and pulmonary embolism (PE) are nonspecific, and their clinical diagnosis is, therefore, unreliable.

NONSURGICAL PATIENTS
See **Medical patients**.

N

NONTHROMBOTIC

DVT is the commonest source of PE. Many nonthrombotic vascular sources e.g. septic, fat, air, tumour, amniotic fluid and foreign bodies can also cause PE.

NORTH AMERICA

A reported 600,000 patients are hospitalized for DVT and 200,000 deaths occur due to VTE in the United States every year.

O

OBESE

Obesity (high body mass index [**BMI**]) is a risk factor for venous thromboembolism (VTE). In obese (BMI >30 kg/m^2) patients, the odds ratio (OR) for deep vein thrombosis (DVT) is 2–3. Patients with waist circumference >100 cm have a four-fold increase in the risk of VTE.

In obese patients, the dose of anticoagulants should be calculated on the basis of total body weight (TBW) and can be administered in two divided doses.

Also, the diagnosis of DVT and pulmonary embolism (PE) is difficult in obese patients.

OBSTETRIC HISTORY

Women with a history of spontaneous abortion, premature birth or stillbirth have a high risk of VTE.

OCCULT

1. About 10% of patients with **idiopathic** DVT have an occult **cancer**.
2. VTE may be the first manifestation of a cancer.

OCP (ORAL CONTRACEPTIVE PILLS)

Oral contraceptive pills (**OCPs**) containing **oestrogen** increase the risk of VTE and should be discontinued 4 weeks before an elective surgery. The couple should be counseled about alternative methods of contraception!

OEDEMA

Pedal oedema may not be present in all cases with DVT, as DVT may occur in one or a few of the many calf veins, allowing venous return through the remaining patent vessels. On the other hand, the presence of pedal oedema does not make a diagnosis of DVT, as the oedema can be caused by several other conditions.

OESTROGEN

Oestrogen-containing **OCPs** and hormone replacement therapy (**HRT**) increase the risk of VTE and should be stopped 4–6 weeks before an elective operation.

OPERATION

Surgical patients are at a higher risk of developing VTE. About 20–25 million surgical procedures are performed in the United States every year. They form a large denominator for the occurrence of VTE.

OR (ODDS RATIO)

The OR of a risk factor for DVT is classified as:

- Strong >10
- Moderate 2–9
- Low <2

ORAL ANTICOAGULANTS

New oral anticoagulants (**NOA** or **NOAC**) e.g. **dabigatran (anti-IIa)**, **apixaban**, **edoxaban** and **rivaroxaban (anti-Xa)**. **Ximelagatran (melagatran)** has been withdrawn from clinical use due to hepatic toxicity.

ORAL ANTICOAGULATION

For the treatment of VTE, oral anticoagulation should **overlap** with parenteral anticoagulation on days 2–5 and should replace parenteral anticoagulation after about 5 days. Some of the newer direct oral anticoagulants (**DOAC**s), however, do not need **bridge therapy** with heparin.

ORAL CONTRACEPTIVE PILLS (OCPs)

See **OCP**.

ORTHOPAEDIC SURGERY

VTE is common after major orthopaedic surgery e.g. hip replacement (**arthroplasty**), knee replacement (arthroplasty), hip fracture surgery (**HFS**), spinal cord injury (**SCI**), etc. Almost all these patients are at high risk for VTE, and thromboprophylaxis is indicated in most of these patients. Some may even need **extended** prophylaxis.

OSTEOPENIA

Osteopenia (reduction in bone density) causing **osteoporosis** is a complication of long-term administration of heparin.

OSTEOPOROSIS

Osteoporosis, as a result of **osteopenia** (reduction in bone density), is a complication of long-term administration of heparin.

OUTPATIENT

1. Prophylaxis for VTE should start at the first outpatient visit of the patient, when advice should be given about stopping **smoking**, discontinuation of oral contraceptive pills (**OCPs**) and hormone replacement therapy (**HRT**) and **ambulation**.
2. Even outpatient treatment of DVT with low-molecular-weight heparin (LMWH) is effective and safe in selected patients.
3. In patients requiring **extended** prophylaxis, LMWH can be administered on an outpatient basis without the need for **monitoring** of the **coagulation profile**.

OVERLAP

An overlap of 5 days is required when changing from injectable (**heparin**) to oral (**warfarin**) anticoagulants.

See **Bridge therapy** also.

P

PAH (PULMONARY ARTERIAL HYPERTENSION)
Chronic recurrent venous thromboembolism (VTE) may cause pulmonary arterial hypertension (PAH) presenting as shortness of breath (SoB) on activity.

PAINFUL
Severe and extensive **iliofemoral** venous thrombosis can result in a pale, swollen and painful leg.

See **Phlegmasia alba dolens** also.

PANCREAS
Cancer is a risk factor for VTE. Patients with **cancer** of the pancreas are at a four to seven times higher risk of VTE as compared to other cancers.

PARADOXICAL EMBOLISM
Embolus from a venous thrombus can enter the arterial circulation through a patent foramen ovale (present in about 30% of the population) and cause systemic embolism e.g. myocardial infarction (**MI**), **stroke** and peripheral arterial occlusion.

PARALYSIS
Patients with paralysis, especially **quadriplegia** or **paraplegia**, have a high risk of VTE.

PARAPLEGIA
Patients with paraplegia due to **stroke** or spinal cord injury (**SCI**) have a high risk of VTE.

PARNAPARIN
Parnaparin is one of the low-molecular-weight heparins (LMWHs). Molecular weight is 4,500 Da, half-life is 6.0 hours and **anti-Xa** to **anti-IIa** ratio is 4.0.

Dose for prophylaxis of VTE is 3,200 IU SC OD.

Dose for treatment of VTE is 4,250 IU SC OD.

PAST HISTORY
Past history of deep vein thrombosis/pulmonary embolism (DVT/PE) increases the risk of VTE – it carries 3 points in the **Caprini** score.

P

PCD (PNEUMATIC COMPRESSION DEVICE)
See **IPC**.

PCDT
Pharmaco-mechanical **catheter-directed thrombolysis (CDT)**.

PE (PULMONARY EMBOLISM)
PE is the most dreaded complication of DVT.

PEGASUS STUDY
Fondaparinux (synthetic factor Xa inhibitor) 2.5. mg SC OD started 6 hours after surgery was found to be noninferior and as safe as **dalteparin** 5,000 IU SC for 5–9 days in a double-blind, randomized trial of 2,858 high-risk patients undergoing abdominal surgery. There were lesser VTE rates in the fondaparinux group (4.6%) vs. the dalteparin group (6.1%). Major bleeding rates were similar (3.4% vs. 2.4%).

Agnelli G, Bergqvist D, Cohen AT, Gallus AS, Gent M; PEGASUS investigators. Randomized clinical trial of postoperative fondaparinux versus perioperative dalteparin for prevention of venous thromboembolism in high-risk abdominal surgery. *Br J Surg*. 2005;92(10):1212–20. doi: 10.1002/bjs.5154

PELVIC FRACTURE
Patients with pelvic fracture are at a high risk for VTE.

PELVIC SURGERY
Pelvic surgery (gastrointestinal, **gynaecological** and urological) is a major risk factor for VTE.

PELVIC TUMOUR
A pelvic tumour may compress the iliac veins and produce venous stasis predisposing to DVT.

PENTAMAKS
Pentasaccharide (fondaparinux 2.5. mg SC OD) (*n* = 361) reduced the incidence of VTE (from 27.8% to 12.5%) as compared to **enoxaparin** 30 mg SC BD (*n* = 363) in a double-blind, randomized study of patients undergoing major knee surgery.

Bauer KA, Eriksson BI, Lassen MR, Turpie AG; Steering Committee of the Pentasaccharide in Major Knee Surgery Study. Fondaparinux compared with enoxaparin for the prevention of venous thromboembolism after elective major knee surgery. *N Engl J Med*. 2001;345(18):1305–10. doi: 10.1056/NEJMoa011099

PENTASACCHARIDE
The pentasaccharide chain in the heparins binds to and activates **antithrombin**. **Fondaparinux** is a synthetic pentasaccharide.

PENTHIFRA (PENTASACCHARIDE IN HIP FRACTURE)

Fondaparinux ($n = 626$) was associated with less VTE (8.3% vs. 19.1%) than **enoxaparin** ($n = 624$) in a double-blind study of patients undergoing hip fracture surgery (**HFS**).

Eriksson BI, Bauer KA, Lassen MR, Turpie AG; Steering Committee of the Pentasaccharide in Hip-Fracture Surgery Study. Fondaparinux compared with enoxaparin for the prevention of venous thromboembolism after hip-fracture surgery. *N Engl J Med.* 2001;345(18):1298–304. doi: 10.1056/NEJMoa011100. PMID: 11794148.

PENTHIFRA-PLUS

In a double-blind, multicentre trial, extended (4 weeks) prophylaxis with **fondaparinux** 2.5 mg in 656 patients undergoing **HFS** reduced the incidence of VTE from 35% to 1.4% and of symptomatic VTE from 2.7% to 0.3%, respectively, as compared to 1-week prophylaxis.

Eriksson BI, Lassen MR; PENTasaccharide in HIp-FRActure Surgery Plus Investigators. Duration of prophylaxis against venous thromboembolism with fondaparinux after hip fracture surgery: A multicenter, randomized, placebo-controlled, double-blind study. *Arch Intern Med.* 2003;163(11): 1337–42. doi: 10.1001/archinte.163.11.1337. PMID: 12796070.

PEPPER

PEPPER is a large proposed clinical trial to address DVT and PE prevention after total hip arthroplasty (**THA**) and total knee arthroplasty (**TKA**) replacement. The following three prophylaxis methods, supported and endorsed by the American College of Chest Physicians (**ACCP**) and the American Academy of Orthopedic Surgeons (**AAOS**) (representing current orthopaedic practice in North America for more than 80% of all hip and knee replacements), will be studied

1. Enteric-coated **aspirin** (regimen with the lowest bleeding risk)
2. Low-intensity (international normalized ratio [**INR**] target 2.0) **warfarin** (low i.e. 1–2% bleeding risk)
3. **Rivaroxaban**, a new oral (direct) factor Xa inhibitor (regimen with a higher i.e. 3–5% bleeding risk)

Prophylaxis will continue for 30 days.
https://clinicaltrials.gov/ct2/show/NCT02810704

PERC (PULMONARY EMBOLISM RULE-OUT CRITERIA)

The Pulmonary Embolism Rule-out Criteria (PERC) include:

Age >50 years, heart rate >100/minute, oxygen saturation (SpO_2) <95%, unilateral leg swelling, haemoptysis, recent (within 4 weeks) trauma or major surgery, previous VTE, hormone use – each is given 1 point.

If the pretest probability (**PTP**) of PE is low (<15%) and the PERC score is 0, the probability of PE is <2% i.e. it is virtually ruled out and no further workup is required.

PERC should not be used if the PTP of PE is moderate or high; **D-dimer** should be done in those cases.

PERFUSION LUNG SCAN

High-probability isotope perfusion lung scan (Fig. P1) is an indication for CT pulmonary angiography (**CTPA**) for confirming the diagnosis of PE.

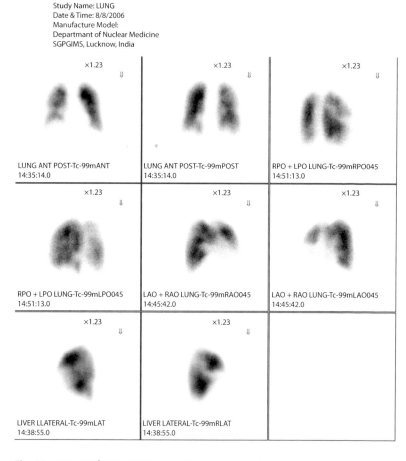

Study Name: LUNG
Date & Time: 8/8/2006
Manufacture Model:
Departmant of Nuclear Medicine
SGPGIMS, Lucknow, India

×1.23

LUNG ANT POST-Tc-99mANT
14:35:14.0

×1.23

LUNG ANT POST-Tc-99mPOST
14:35:14.0

×1.23

RPO + LPO LUNG-Tc-99mRPO045
14:51:13.0

×1.23

RPO + LPO LUNG-Tc-99mLPO045
14:51:13.0

×1.23

LAO + RAO LUNG-Tc-99mRAO045
14:45:42.0

×1.23

LAO + RAO LUNG-Tc-99mLAO045
14:45:42.0

×1.23

LIVER LLATERAL-Tc-99mLAT
14:38:55.0

×1.23

LIVER LATERAL-Tc-99mRLAT
14:38:55.0

Fig. P1   Lung perfusion isotope scan is a noninvasive investigation for the diagnosis of PE.

PERSISTENT

Risk factors for VTE may be transient or persistent. Persistent risk factors for VTE include reversible conditions e.g. curable malignancy, inflammatory bowel disease (**IBD**), etc., and irreversible conditions e.g. inheritable **thrombophilia**s, chronic heart failure (**CHF**), and metastatic end-stage **cancer**.

PESI (PULMONARY EMBOLISM SEVERITY INDEX)

The Pulmonary Embolism Severity Index (PESI) (Table P1) predicts the 30-day outcome of patients with PE using clinical criteria viz. age, sex, history of **cancer**, history of congestive heart failure (**CHF**), history of chronic lung disease, heart rate >110, BP <100 mm Hg, respiratory rate >30, temperature <36° C, altered mental status, O_2 saturation <90%.

Table P1   Pulmonary Embolism Severity Index (PESI)

Class	PESI score	30-day mortality %
I	0–65	0.0–1.6
II	66–85	1.7–3.5
III	86–105	3.2–7.1
IV	106–125	4.0–11.4
V	>125	10.0–24.5

Source: https://www.mdcalc.com/pulmonary-embolism-severity-index-pesi

PFS (PREFILLED SYRINGE)

Fine (27 gauge) needle, automatic needle protection system, including a security sleeve which covers the used needle after injection and thus minimizes the risk of needle stick injuries; it also prevents reuse of the disposable syringe.

PGIMER (POST-GRADUATE INSTITUTE OF MEDICAL EDUCATION AND RESEARCH)

Post-Graduate Institute of Medical Education and Research (PGIMER), Chandigarh, India

From 1997 to 2004, autopsies were conducted in 1,000 adult medical patients. PE was found in 159, it was fatal in 36, it made a significant contribution to death in 90 and it was incidental in 33. PE was suspected clinically in only 30%, diagnosed antemortem in only 10% and 80% of patients with PE were young (<50 years). Sepsis was present in 32% and **cancer** in 17% of patients with fatal PE.

See **Autopsy** also.

Kakkar N, Vasishta RK. Pulmonary embolism in medical patients: An autopsy-based study. *Clin Appl Thromb Hemost.* 2008;14(2):159–67. doi: 10.1177/1076029607308389. Epub 2007 Dec 26. PMID: 18160596.

PHARMACOLOGICAL

Pharmacological thromboprophylaxis with anticoagulants is more effective than mechanical methods of thromboprophylaxis.

PHENINDIONE

Phenindione is a vitamin K antagonist (**VKA**). It is not used because of a high risk of hypersensitivity reaction. **Warfarin**, another VKA, is preferred.

PHLEBOGRAPHY

Invasive phlebography (**venography**) is now rarely used for the diagnosis of DVT; it has largely been replaced by **Doppler** ultrasound (US).

PHLEGMASIA ALBA DOLENS

Commonly seen with **pregnancy** or **puerperium**-related DVT; more common in patients with **cancer**

Caused by a **massive** DVT in the iliofemoral veins and distal veins associated with vasospasm. Clinical features include pain, blanching and oedema. It results in a chronically swollen leg – sometimes with ulceration – and may progress to **phlegmasia cerulea dolens**.

Frequently, iliofemoral thrombosis is associated with **May Thurner syndrome**. This is more common on the left side and remains undiagnosed until the patient develops DVT, particularly during **pregnancy**.

PHLEGMASIA CERULEA DOLENS

May be preceded by **phlegmasia alba dolens** – extremely painful, blue (cyanotic), massively swollen leg. This is a limb-threatening condition, as it may cause venous gangrene due to compartment syndrome and arterial insufficiency requiring even amputation; it may even be fatal. It is a vascular emergency requiring **thrombolysis** or **thrombectomy**.

PLASTER CAST

Immobilization (>1 month) due to the application of a plaster cast to a lower limb increases the risk of DVT.

PLATELET

1. No anticoagulation should be given if platelet count is <50,000.
2. Platelet counts should be checked 2–3 days after starting heparin; heparin should be stopped if platelet counts are <100,000 because of the risk of heparin-induced thrombocytopenia (**HIT**).

PLETHYSMOGRAPHY

Impedance plethysmography (IPG) records electrical impedance in the calf following temporary compression occlusion of the proximal veins by applying a cuff in the thigh. IPG, however, is not a sensitive or specific investigation for the diagnosis of DVT and is no longer used.

POLYTRAUMA

Patients with polytrauma, especially those with **hip fracture** or **pelvic fracture**, are at a high risk to develop VTE.

PORCINE ORIGIN

Heparins are of porcine origin. Their use may have religious and cultural implications in some patients with strong beliefs.

PORTAL VEIN

Patients with **thrombophilic** disorders may develop thrombosis in the portal vein (Fig. P2a), which may extend proximally into the superior **mesenteric** vein (SMV) (Fig. P2b), the splenic vein (Fig. P2c) and distally to one of the branches of the portal vein (Fig. P2d). Acute portal vein thrombosis may cause ischemic gangrene of the bowel, but chronic thrombosis may remain largely **asymptomatic (silent)** because of the development of collateral venous channels around the thrombosed vein (Fig. P3).

POSITION

Position of the patient during an operation is very important; an incorrect position during surgery may cause venous compression and stasis and lead to DVT (and nerve injury). The **lithotomy** position also increases the risk of VTE.

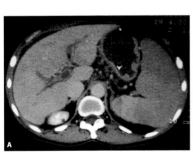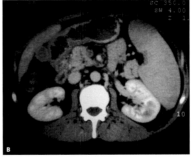

Fig. P2   Thrombus (hypodense) a. in the main portal vein (MPV), extending into b. the superior mesenteric vein (SMV), c. splenic vein and d. right portal vein. (*Continued*)

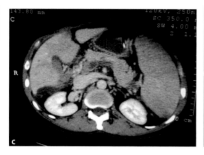
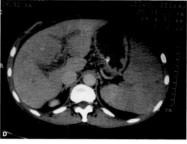

Fig. P2 (Cont.)   Thrombus (hypodense) a. in the main portal vein (MPV), extending into b. the superior mesenteric vein (SMV), c. splenic vein and d. right portal vein.

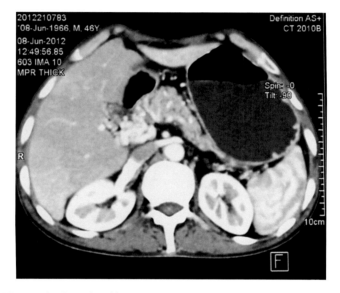

Fig. P3   Portal vein replaced by cavernoma i.e. a bunch of collaterals. Inferior vena cava (IVC) also shows a thrombus at the site of joining of the renal veins.

POSTOPERATIVE

Patients who undergo an operation are at a higher risk of developing VTE. Postoperative risk of VTE is maximum during 3–7 days after surgery.

POSTPARTUM

The increased risk of VTE during **pregnancy** continues after the delivery for 4–6 weeks in the postpartum period; VTE prophylaxis, if indicated and started during the **pregnancy**, should, therefore, be continued in the postpartum period also for 3–6 weeks.

Bates SM, Middeldorp S, Rodger M, James AH, Greer I. Guidance for the treatment and prevention of obstetric-associated venous thromboembolism. *J Thromb Thrombolysis.* 2016;41(1):92–128. doi: 10.1007/s11239-015-1309-0

PPS (POSTPHLEBITIC SYNDROME)

Postphlebitic syndrome (PPS) is a disabling long-term **sequelae** of DVT. It results in a chronically swollen leg, sometimes with ulceration, causing complete obstruction of the venous outflow. It can be prevented by using graduated compression stockings (**GCS**) after DVT; they should be started within 1month of DVT, and have to be used for 1 year or even longer.

See **PTS** also.

PREDICT

A large number of patients may have **risk factors** for VTE, but it is not possible to predict which of these patients will go on to develop VTE; hence, prophylaxis is important.

PREGNANCY

Pregnancy is associated with a physiological hypercoagulable state due to an increase in the procoagulants and impaired fibrinolysis. Pregnant women have a four to five times higher risk of VTE. PE is a leading cause of maternal peripartum deaths in the developed world (Confidential Enquiries into Maternal and Child Health [CEMACH], UK). This risk is more in older (>35 years) women, those with preeclampsia and those undergoing caesarean section.

D-dimer is not useful either for diagnosis or exclusion of VTE, as the levels are normally high during pregnancy; imaging should instead be used.

Iliofemoral DVT is more common during pregnancy than calf DVT. DVT of pregnancy is associated with vasospasm leading to **phlegmasia alba dolens**. Pregnant women at high risk of DVT should receive anticoagulation prophylaxis during pregnancy and for up to 6 weeks postpartum. Pregnant women at low risk of DVT may be given anticoagulants only postpartum.

Warfarin crosses the placenta and may cause embryopathy, foetal bleeding and spontaneous abortion and is contraindicated antenatally; unfractionated heparin (UFH) and LMWH are preferred but should be discontinued 24 hours before labour/caesarean section. Warfarin is not secreted in breast milk and can be used by the lactating mother postnatally.

PREVALENCE

DVT is common in hospitalized patients. DVT occurred in about 20% and PE in about 1–2% of patients undergoing surgery without prophylaxis. About 23 million operations are performed every year in the United States. In the absence of thromboprophylaxis, calf (distal) DVT may occur in 40–80%, proximal DVT in

10–20% and PE in 5–10% of patients undergoing major orthopaedic surgery (hip and knee **arthroplasty**, hip fracture surgery [**HFS**].

DVT can occur in 60–80% of patients with spinal cord injury (**SCI**); 20–40% of patients with **stroke**; 15–40% of patients undergoing major general, **gynaecological**, urologic or neurosurgery; and 10–20% of medical patients.

PREVENT (PREVENTION OF RECURRENT VENOUS THROMBOEMBOLISM) STUDY

Recurrent VTE was less common ($n = 14$ vs. 37) in the low-intensity **warfarin** (INR 1.5–2.0) group ($n = 255$) than in the placebo group ($n = 253$).

Ridker PM, Goldhaber SZ, Danielson E, Rosenberg Y, Eby CS, Deitcher SR, Cushman M, Moll S, Kessler CM, Elliott CG, Paulson R, Wong T, Bauer KA, Schwartz BA, Miletich JP, Bounameaux H, Glynn RJ; PREVENT Investigators. Long-term, low-intensity warfarin therapy for the prevention of recurrent venous thromboembolism. *N Engl J Med.* 2003;348(15):1425–34. doi: 10.1056/NEJMoa035029. Epub 2003 Feb 24. PMID: 12601075.

PREVENT

Dalteparin 5,000 IU/day vs. placebo in a randomized, double-blind, multicentre, placebo-controlled trial of 3,706 general medical patients (VTE 2.8% vs. 5.0%).

Leizorovicz A, Cohen AT, Turpie AG, Olsson CG, Vaitkus PT, Goldhaber SZ; PREVENT Medical Thromboprophylaxis Study Group. Randomized, placebo-controlled trial of dalteparin for the prevention of venous thromboembolism in acutely ill medical patients. *Circulation.* 2004;110(7):874–79. doi: 10.1161/01.CIR.0000138928.83266.24. Epub 2004 Aug 2. PMID: 15289368.

PREVENTABLE

DVT and PE are preventable causes of mortality and morbidity. PE is the most common preventable cause of death in hospitalized patients.

PREVENTION

Prophylaxis, timely diagnosis and appropriate management of DVT can prevent PE to a great extent.

PREVIOUS

A previous episode of VTE is a high-risk factor for future VTE.

PRINCE (PROPHYLAXIS IN INTERNAL MEDICINE WITH ENOXAPARIN)

Multicentre, controlled, randomized, open study in which patients received either **enoxaparin** (40 mg once daily) or UFH (5,000 IU three times daily) for

10 +/– 2 days in 655 patients in 64 medical departments in Germany. VTE events were 8.4% vs. 10.4%.

Kleber FX, Witt C, Vogel G, Koppenhagen K, Schomaker U, Flosbach CW; THE-PRINCE Study Group. Randomized comparison of enoxaparin with unfractionated heparin for the prevention of venous thromboembolism in medical patients with heart failure or severe respiratory disease. *Am Heart J.* 2003;145(4):614–21. doi: 10.1067/mhj.2003.189. PMID: 12679756.

PROBABILITY
Several scores are used to test the probability of VTE. If the pretest probability (**PTP**) of DVT is unlikely, **D-dimer** should be done. If D-dimer is negative, there is no DVT; no further tests are required.

If the **PTP** of DVT is likely or if D-dimer is positive, US should be done to detect DVT.

PROGNOSIS
The prognosis of patients with **cancer** who have had an episode of VTE is worse than that of those without VTE.

PROPHYLAXIS
DVT prophylaxis is the most appropriate strategy. This includes **screening**, assessment and implementation of prophylaxis. Prophylaxis includes **mechanical** and **pharmacological** methods. Prophylaxis is easier than treatment; also, it is effective, as it decreases the risk of VTE.

PROPAGATE
Without treatment, about 20–25% of distal (calf) DVTs propagate to **proximal** (iliofemoral) veins.

PROTAMINE
Protamine sulphate is very useful to neutralize the effect of UFH in case of serious bleeding. One mg of protamine neutralizes 100 IU of UFH. Protamine should be administered as a slow intravenous (IV) infusion.

The therapeutic effect of LMWH is only partly reversed by protamine. Protamine reverses the **antithrombin** activity of LMWH but not its anti–factor X activity. One mg of protamine neutralizes 1 mg of **enoxaparin**; if the last dose of enoxaparin was given 8 hours ago, the full dose of protamine (1 mg for 1 mg) may be used; a half-dose of protamine (0.5 mg for 1 mg enoxaparin) may be used if the last dose of enoxaparin was given 8–12 hours ago.

PROTECHT
Nadroparin reduced the risk of VTE in ambulatory **cancer** patients receiving **chemotherapy**.

P

Agnelli G, Gussoni G, Bianchini C, Verso M, Mandalà M, Cavanna L, Barni S, Labianca R, Buzzi F, Scambia G, Passalacqua R, Ricci S, Gasparini G, Lorusso V, Bonizzoni E, Tonato M; PROTECHT Investigators. Nadroparin for the prevention of thromboembolic events in ambulatory patients with metastatic or locally advanced solid cancer receiving chemotherapy: A randomised, placebo-controlled, double-blind study. *Lancet Oncol.* 2009;10(10):943–49. doi: 10.1016/S1470-2045(09)70232-3. Epub 2009 Aug 31. PMID: 19726226.

PROTEINS C AND S

Proteins C and S are vitamin K dependent plasma proteins that play a role in anti-coagulation. Deficiency of proteins **C** and **S** (also known as **antithrombin 3**) results in a **thrombophilic** state and increases the risk of VTE. These patients are prone to have **recurrent** VTE and may require long-term, even life-long, anticoagulation.

PROTHROMBIN

Prothrombin (factor II) is converted to **thrombin** (factor IIa) by factor Xa. This is an important step in the **coagulation cascade**.

PROTHROMBIN GENE

Prothrombin (factor II) is an important component of the **coagulation cascade**. A mutation of the prothrombin gene increases the risk of VTE.

PROVE STUDY (LEE. *J THROMB HEMOST* 2005)

Prospective registry on VTE events – 19 countries, 254 centres, 3,526 patients. Both proximal and calf DVT was seen in 52%, calf DVT in 24% and proximal DVT in 18% patients. In 1,126 patients from Europe and Australia, calf DVT was seen in 40% and proximal DVT in 12%. In 1,695 patients from Asia, calf DVT was seen in 12% and proximal DVT in 22%. In 667 patients from India, both proximal and calf DVT was seen in 54%, calf DVT in 13% and proximal DVT in 17%. Only 7% of patients in India received prophylaxis.

PROVOKED DVT

DVT occurring after some provocation e.g. prolonged lying down, long operation, etc. (cf. **unprovoked** DVT).

PROXIMAL DVT

The majority of proximal (**iliofemoral**) DVTs occur as a result of the propagation of the distal (calf) DVT, but about one-quarter to one-third of the thrombi in the lower limbs may start in the proximal veins. Thrombi in the proximal veins are more likely to result in PE as compared to those in the distal (calf) veins.

PT (PROTHROMBIN TIME)

Prothrombin time (PT) and international normalized ratio (**INR**) need to be monitored if the patient is on therapeutic doses of **warfarin**. Direct oral anticoagulants (**DOACs**), however, do not need PT/INR monitoring.

PTP (PRE-TEST PROBABILITY)

Clinical PTP of DVT using various scores e.g. **Caprini**, **Wells**, is classified as high, intermediate and low.

PTS (POST-THROMBOTIC SYNDROME)

Post-thrombotic syndrome (PTS) is caused by persistent venous occlusion/venous valvular incompetence. It results in chronic leg swelling, pain, dermatitis, discoloration, itching and ulceration. About 30% of patients with DVT will develop PTS in the long term. PTS is a permanent disability. It is estimated that about 15 million people suffer from PTS in the United States; this results in a loss of about 2 million workdays every year (Nicolaides. *Int Angiol* 2001). About 4% of patients will develop a **venous ulcer** over a period of 20 years after an episode of DVT. Use of **GCS** can reduce the risk of PTS. They should be started within 1 month of DVT and used for 1–2 years.

Nicolaides AN, Breddin HK, Fareed J, Goldhaber S, Haas S, Hull R, Kalodiki E, Myers K, Samama M, Sasahara A; Cardiovascular Disease Educational and Research Trust and the International Union of Angiology. Prevention of venous thromboembolism. International Consensus Statement. Guidelines compiled in accordance with the scientific evidence. *Int Angiol.* 2001;20(1):1–37. PMID: 11342993.

PUBLIC HEALTH

VTE is a major public health issue, as it carries high morbidity and mortality, though it is easily prevented.

PUERPERAL CVT (CEREBRAL VENOUS THROMBOSIS)

Pregnant women are prone to developing cerebral venous thrombosis (CVT) due to a temporary reversible hypercoagulable state in **pregnancy**. Puerperal CVT is more common in Indian women. It is treated with heparin for up to 2–3 weeks after delivery.

PULMONARY ANGIOGRAPHY, CONVENTIONAL

Conventional (invasive) pulmonary angiography, earlier the gold standard for diagnosing PE, is being replaced by **CTPA** (Fig. P4) or MR pulmonary angiography (**MRPA**). It shows an intraluminal filling defect or abrupt cutoff in the pulmonary artery (Fig. P5) in the presence of PE.

PULMONARY EMBOLECTOMY

Rarely, an emergency pulmonary embolectomy may have to be performed in a patient with a **massive** PE who is hemodynamically unstable in whom **thrombolysis**

P

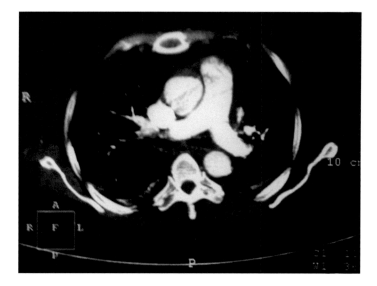

Fig. P4   Pulmonary angiography (CTPA or MRPA) is the investigation of choice for the diagnosis of PE.

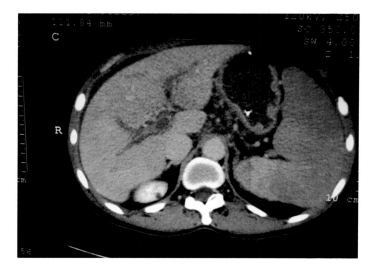

Fig. P5   Pulmonary angiography (CTPA) shows emboli in the right and left pulmonary arteries and their branches. (Image courtesy Dr Shivani Rao, Indira Gandhi Medical College, Shimla.)

is contraindicated or has failed. Mortality, however, is very high: 20–40%. Pulmonary embolectomy can be done percutaneously using a suction/fragmentation device.

PULMONARY EMBOLISM (PE)

APE is the most severe complication of DVT; it can occur in the absence of DVT also. **Proximal** (**iliofemoral**) DVT is associated with a higher risk of PE than distal (calf) DVT.

PE results in impaired gas exchange because of poor perfusion caused by vasoconstriction due to the release of inflammatory mediators e.g. serotonin in the lungs, hypoxemia due to intrapulmonary shunting of blood and atelectasis.

PE manifests as breathlessness of sudden onset, chest pain, discomfort or tightness and/or haemoptysis. Signs include tachypnoea, tachycardia, hypotension (systolic blood pressure [BP]<90 mm Hg), hypoxia; the lungs, however, may be clear on auscultation.

Acute PE occurred in about 1% of 51,645 hospitalized patients; it caused or contributed to death in 3% of cases (Stein. *Chest* 1995). PE is the sole or the major cause of 10% of acute adult deaths in hospitals; it is the most common preventable cause of in-hospital death. The majority of patients who have a fatal PE are medical (nonsurgical) patients. PE is the third most common (after coronary artery disease [CAD] and **stroke**) cardiovascular cause of death.

Diagnosis of PE can be suspected on V/Q scan, **CTPA**, MRPA, echocardiography. Most cases of PE can be managed with anticoagulation; **thrombolysis** is required in patients with **massive** PE with hemodynamic instability. Rarely, **embolectomy** (**surgical thrombectomy**) may be required.

Stein PD, Henry JW. Prevalence of acute pulmonary embolism among patients in a general hospital and at autopsy. *Chest.* 1995;108(4):978–81. doi: 10.1378/chest.108.4.978. PMID: 7555172.

PULMONARY ARTERIAL HYPERTENSION

VTE can cause chronic thromboembolic pulmonary arterial hypertension manifesting as shortness of breath (SoB) in the long term.

Q

QUADRIPLEGIA

Patients with quadriplegia due to **stroke** or spinal cord injury (**SCI**) have a high risk of venous thromboembolism (VTE).

QUALITY OF LIFE

Acute VTE results in significant morbidity and may even cause mortality. **Sequelae** of VTE i.e. post-thrombotic syndrome (**PTS**) can interfere with the quality of life (QoL) of patients.

QUESTIONNAIRE

There are several ways to evaluate the risk of VTE in the patients. A medical history questionnaire may be administered to the patients to evaluate their risk for VTE.

R

RACE

Race (ethnicity) is an important determinant of the risk of VTE. The risk of venous thromboembolism (VTE) is more in African Americans than in **Asians**.

RADIONUCLIDE VENOGRAPHY WITH PULMONARY SCINTIGRAPHY

Isotope scintigraphy is a less invasive (but at the same time less accurate) test for the diagnosis of deep vein thrombosis/pulmonary embolism (DVT-PE).

Sir Ganga Ram Hospital, New Delhi India: In 1,552 patients with clinically suspected lower limb DVT, radionuclide venography detected DVT in 744 patients (521, 70% suprapopliteal); 294 out of 744 (40%) showed a high-probability isotope lung scan for PE (but 47% of these had no clinical manifestation of PE).

Parakh R, Kapadia SR, Sen I, Agarwal S, Grover T, Yadav A. Pulmonary embolism: A frequent occurrence in Indian patients with symptomatic lower limb venous thrombosis. *Asian J Surg.* 2006;29(2):86–91. doi: 10.1016/S1015-9584(09)60113-5. PMID: 16644508.

RATIONALE

VTE prophylaxis is based on the facts that VTE is common, can be dangerous (even fatal) and can be easily prevented.

RCOG (ROYAL COLLEGE OF OBSTETRICIANS AND GYNAECOLOGISTS)

The Royal College of Obstetricians and Gynaecologists (RCOG) guidelines for thromboprophylaxis in **pregnancy** and puerperium.

https://www.rcog.org.uk/globalassets/documents/guidelines/gtg-37a.pdf

RCT (RANDOMIZED CONTROLLED TRIAL)

Randomized controlled trials (RCTs) allocate the subjects randomly to the study and the control groups in order to eliminate any selection bias and produce the highest level of evidence.

REASONS

There are several reasons for the **underutilization** of VTE. Common reasons for not using VTE thromboprophylaxis are lack of awareness, fear of **bleeding** and extra costs.

RECANALIZATION

DVT causes blockage of the veins due to the thrombus. Recanalization of thrombosed blocked veins can occur after spontaneous natural fibrinolysis of the thrombus.

RECOMMENDATION, LEVELS OF

- *Level A:* Evidence class I or overwhelming evidence class II – high degree of clinical certainty
- *Level B:* Evidence class II or strong consensus on evidence class III – moderate degree of clinical certainty
- *Level C:* Panel consensus – preliminary, inconclusive, conflicting evidence

RECURRENCE

In a systematic review and meta-analysis of 18 studies involving 7,515 patients with a first **unprovoked** VTE event who had completed at least 3 months of treatment, the risk of **recurrent** VTE was 10% in the first year after treatment, 16% at 2 years, 25% at 5 years, and 36% at 10 years, with 4% of recurrent VTE events resulting in death.

The risk of recurrent DVT is higher (about 20% within 6 months) in patients with **cancer**.

Khan F, Rahman A, Carrier M, et al. Long term risk of symptomatic recurrent venous thromboembolism after discontinuation of anticoagulant treatment for first unprovoked venous thromboembolism event: systematic review and meta-analysis. *BMJ*. 2019;366:l4363. doi: 10.1136/bmj.l4363

RECURRENT DVT

Patients with DVT, especially those with a nonmodifiable risk factor e.g. **cancer**, are at a high risk for a recurrent DVT. The recurrence rate may be as high as 25% within 5 years and 33% in 10 years. However, the risk is maximum in the first 6–12 months. Recurrent VTE occurred in 7% of patients with DVT in 6 months. Recurrent VTE is more likely to occur in patients with **idiopathic** VTE (no cause found) than in those with VTE due to a known cause. Recurrent VTE can be prevented by long-term oral anticoagulation prophylaxis with low-molecular-weight heparin (LMWH) or **warfarin**. Patients with a reversible risk factor e.g. trauma, immobilization, surgery are treated for 3 months; those with no identifiable risk factor, for 6 months; and those with an irreversible risk factor e.g. cancer, for 6–12 months.

Recurrent DVT may be an indication for long-term, may be even life-long, anticoagulation.

REGISTRY

Various VTE-related registries e.g. ENDORSE (Epidemiologic International Day for the Evaluation of Patients at Risk of Venous Thrombosis in the Acute Hospital Care Setting – 90,000 patients in 358 hospitals in 32 countries), GLORY (The Global Orthopedic Registry – hip and knee **arthroplasty** in 5,000+ patients from 100 hospitals in 12 countries 2001–2005), RIETE (The RegistroInformatizado de EnfermedadTromboEmbólica – The Computerized Registry of Patients with Venous Thromboembolism with more than 90,000 cases) have the data of a large number of patients.

R

REMOVABLE
The conventional inferior vena cava (IVC) filters were not removable. Removable IVC **filters** are now available.

RENAL DYSFUNCTION
Patients who are at risk to develop DVT or PE often have renal dysfunction. LMWHs are excreted mainly by the kidneys; there is thus a direct relationship between the degree of renal dysfunction and their bioaccumulation. No dose adjustment is required for LMWH in patients with mild (**creatinine clearance** [**CC**] 50–80 mL/minute) and moderate (CC 30–50 mL/minute) renal dysfunction. These patients, however, should be carefully observed for bleeding. In patients with severe (CC <30 mL/minute) renal dysfunction, a 30 mg (i.e. 50%) dose of **enoxaparin** should be used for prophylaxis or else unfractionated heparin (UFH) should be used. Higher-molecular-weight LMWHs e.g. **dalteparin** and **tinzaparin** are less dependent on renal clearance and do not need dose modification. They have less risk of accumulation and less risk of bleeding in patients with **renal dysfunction**.

Fondaparinux is contraindicated in patients with renal dysfunction.

Direct oral anticoagulants (**DOAC**s) are contraindicated in patients with severe renal insufficiency; renally adjusted dosing can be used in patients with mild-to-moderate renal impairment.

RESOURCE EXPENDITURE
VTE puts lots of strain on resource expenditure because of sophisticated investigations required for its diagnosis and hospitalized management. VTE prophylaxis is, therefore, a cost-beneficial strategy.

RESPIRATORY MODULATION
Respiratory modulation in the flow velocity in the lower limb veins on Doppler rules out iliocaval venous obstruction.

RHF (RIGHT HEART FAILURE)
Increased pulmonary vascular resistance in PE may result in right heart failure (RHF). These changes will be seen in electrocardiogram (**ECG**) and **echo**.

REVERSAL
In the case of major or significant **bleeding**, the therapeutic effect of UFH can be reversed with **protamine**.

RIGHT ATRIAL THROMBUS
Patients with an indwelling central venous catheter (**CVC**) can develop a right atrial thrombus, which may be a source of PE.

RISK ASSESSMENT

R

All patients admitted to a hospital must be subjected to some assessment of their risk (Fig. R1) for VTE.

A 1-point risk assessment study of 68,183 hospitalized patients all over the world showed that 52% of patients were at risk for VTE (51% of 2,058 Indian patients were at risk) (Cohen. *Lancet* 2008).

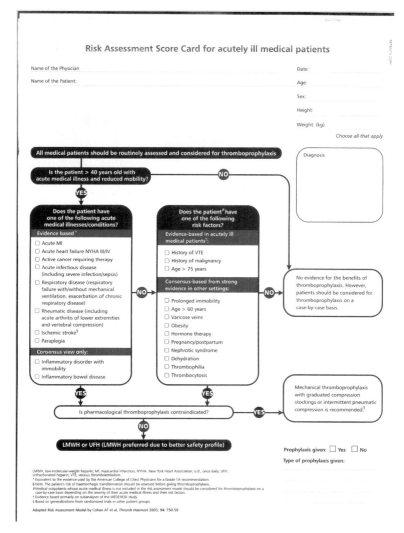

Fig. R1   All patients admitted to a hospital should be assessed for their risk of VTE.

Mandatory risk assessment of all hospitalized patients reduced the risk of post-discharge VTE-related deaths in the UK.

Cohen AT, Tapson VF, Bergmann JF, Goldhaber SZ, Kakkar AK, Deslandes B, Huang W, Zayaruzny M, Emery L, Anderson FA Jr; ENDORSE Investigators. Venous thromboembolism risk and prophylaxis in the acute hospital care setting (ENDORSE study): A multinational cross-sectional study. *Lancet*. 2008;371(9610):387–94. doi: 10.1016/S0140-6736(08)60202-0. Erratum in: *Lancet*. 2008;371(9628):1914. PMID: 18242412.

RISK/BENEFIT RATIO
Thromboprophylaxis has a desirable risk/benefit ratio, as the risk of major (significant) **bleeding** is low and benefit in terms of decrease in incidence of DVT/PE is high.

RISK CATEGORY
Based on the presence or absence of various VTE **risk factors**, a VTE risk score is calculated and, based on this score, patients are stratified into VTE risk groups.

Total VTE risk score	VTE risk category
1	Low
2	Moderate
3–4	High
5 or more	Highest

The risk of DVT, PE and mortality increases with the increasing risk category (Table R1).

Table R1   Risk category and mortality

Level of risk of VTE	Calf DVT	Proximal DVT	Clinical PE	Fatal PE
Low	2%	0.4%	0.2%	Nil
Moderate	10–20%	2–4%	1–2%	0.1–0.4%
High	20–40%	4–8%	2–4%	0.4–1.0%
Highest	40–80%	10–20%	4–10%	0.2–5%

Source: From ACCP *Chest* 2004.

RISK FACTORS
A risk factor for VTE can be personal or clinical, **inherited** or **acquired**, transient or permanent. They could be patient related, disease related or treatment related.

R

Risk factors for VTE include increasing **age, obesity, varicose veins, smoking, pregnancy** and **postpartum** period; acute medical illnesses (congestive heart failure [**CHF**], respiratory failure, **stroke**, nephrotic syndrome); **cancer**; major or lower extremity **trauma**; prolonged immobility; prolonged pelvic or lower limb surgery; chemotherapy or radiotherapy; previous VTE; oestrogen-containing oral contraceptive pills (**OCPs**); hormone replacement therapy (**HRT**); central venous catheter (**CVC**) placement; and many others.

Most hospitalized patients have one or more risk factors for VTE. In one study about 40% of hospitalized patients were found to have three or more risk factors for VTE. The prevalence of risk factors in 1,231 patients treated for acute VTE was age >40 years (89%), obesity (38%), previous VTE (26%), cancer (22%), bed rest >5 days (12%) and major surgery (11%) (Anderson. *Circulation* 2003).

Risk for VTE is cumulative e.g. patients with **hip fracture** are old and patients with **cancer** undergo major surgery, etc.

Five hundred patients admitted to the Department of Surgical Gastroenterology at SGPGIMS – a tertiary care centre at Lucknow in north India – were found to be in the highest (35%), high (33%), moderate (30%) and low (2%) VTE risk category (unpublished data).

Anderson FA Jr, Spencer FA. Risk factors for venous thromboembolism. *Circulation.* 2003;107(23 Suppl 1):I9–16. doi: 10.1161/01.CIR.0000078469.07362.E6. PMID: 12814980.

RISK OF BLEEDING
One of the main reasons for not using VTE thromboprophylaxis is the fear of bleeding. There is, however, no or little increase in significant bleeding with prophylactic doses of UFH, LMWH or vitamin K antagonists (**VKAs**).

RISK OF DVT
The risk of DVT in various groups of patients is as follows: medical patients (10–20%); general surgery, major **gynaecological** surgery, major urologic surgery, **neurosurgery** (15–40%); **stroke** (20–50%); hip or knee replacement surgery, hip fracture surgery (**HFS**) (40–60%); major trauma (40–80%); spinal cord injury (**SCI**) (60–80%); and critical care patients (10–80%) (Geerts. *Chest* 2004).

Geerts WH, Pineo GF, Heit JA, Bergqvist D, Lassen MR, Colwell CW, Ray JG. Prevention of venous thromboembolism: the Seventh ACCP Conference on Antithrombotic and Thrombolytic Therapy. *Chest.* 2004;126(3 Suppl):338S–400S. doi: 10.1378/chest.126.3_suppl.338S. PMID: 15383478.

RISK OF PE
DVT is the precursor of PE. The risk of PE is higher with **proximal** (**iliofemoral**) DVT than with distal (calf) DVT.

RIVAROXABAN

Rivaroxaban is a direct oral anticoagulant (**DOAC**) and a selective factor Xa inhibitor. It is started 6–10 hours after surgery. The dose for prophylaxis is 10 mg OD. The dose for treatment is 15 mg PO BID × 21 days, then 20 mg OD. Dose for prevention of recurrent VTE is 10–20 mg OD. It does not require coagulation monitoring.

The EINSTEIN trials compared rivaroxaban with LMWH. For the treatment of PE, it was noninferior to LMWH.

EINSTEIN–PE Investigators, Büller HR, Prins MH, Lensin AW, Decousus H, Jacobson BF, Minar E, Chlumsky J, Verhamme P, Wells P, Agnelli G, Cohen A, Berkowitz SD, Bounameaux H, Davidson BL, Misselwitz F, Gallus AS, Raskob GE, Schellong S, Segers A. Oral rivaroxaban for the treatment of symptomatic pulmonary embolism. *N Engl J Med*. 2012 Apr 5;366(14):1287–97. doi: 10.1056/NEJMoa1113572. Epub 2012 Mar 26. PMID: 22449293.

ROGERS SCORE

The ninth edition of the American College of Chest Physicians (**ACCP**) Antithrombotic Therapy and Prevention of Thrombosis guidelines (AT9) have recognized only two **risk assessment** tools in the nonorthopaedic surgical population: the Rogers score and the **Caprini** score. The Rogers score is based on variables that were found to be independent predictors of VTE risk such as surgical procedure, female sex and a variety of other individual patient characteristics. Unlike the Caprini score, the Rogers score does not take into account certain VTE risk factors, including any personal or family history of VTE and **thrombophilia**. The Rogers score (Table R2) has been validated in general, vascular and thoracic surgery.

Table R2   Rogers score

Risk factor	Specific risk factor	Score
Operation	Respiratory	9
	Thoracoabdominal aneurysm	7
	Abdominal aneurysm	4
	Mouth, palate	4
	Stomach, intestines	4
	Skin	3
	Hernia	2
American Society of Anesthesiologists (ASA) score	3,4,5	2
	2	1
	1	0

(Continued)

Table R2 Rogers score (*Continued*)

Risk factor	Specific risk factor	Score
Gender	Female	
Work relative value update (RUV)	>17	3
	10–17	2
	<10	0
2-point factors	Disseminated cancer	2
	Chemotherapy within 1 month	2
	Serum sodium >145 mmol/L	2
	Transfusion >4 units within 72 hours of operation	2
	Ventilator	2
1-point factors	Wound class 3 or 4	1
	Hematocrit (Hct) <38	1
	Bilirubin >1.0	1
	Dyspnoea	1
	Albumin <3.5	1
	Emergency	1
Rogers score	Risk category	Observed risk of VTE
<7	Very low	0
7–10	Low	0.7%
>10	Moderate	1.0

ROLLED DOWN

Proper application of graduated compression stockings (**GCS**) is important. Rolled-down GCS may act like a tourniquet and have an adverse effect i.e. caused venous stasis; this should be avoided.

ROYAL COLLEGE OF OBSTETRICIANS AND GYNAECOLOGISTS (RCOG)

See **RCOG**.

S

S (PROTEIN)

Protein S is a vitamin K dependent plasma protein which plays a role in antico-agulation. Protein S (as also **protein C**) deficiency creates a thrombophilic state and increases the risk of venous thromboembolism (VTE).

SAFETY

Thromboprophylaxis to prevent or reduce the risk of VTE is the number-one strategy to improve the safety of patients admitted to hospitals.

SAFETY PROFILE

Low-molecular-weight heparins (LMWHs) have a better safety profile than unfractionated heparin (UFH) in terms of risk of major bleeding.

SAGES (SOCIETY OF AMERICAN GASTROINTESTINAL AND ENDOSCOPIC SURGEONS)

VTE prophylaxis guidelines for laparoscopic surgery.

https://www.sages.org/publications/guidelines/guidelines-for-deep-venous-thrombosis-prophylaxis-during-laparoscopic-surgery/

SCI (SPINAL CORD INJURY)

See **Spinal cord injury**.

SCOTTISH INTERCOLLEGIATE GUIDELINES NETWORK (SIGN)

See **SIGN**.

SCREENING

1. Screening (with **Doppler** ultrasound [US]) of all or at-risk patients for **asymp-tomatic** (**silent**) deep vein thrombosis (DVT) is logistically difficult – it does not prevent pulmonary embolism (PE) and is not cost-effective. Patients at risk of developing VTE should rather receive thromboprophylaxis.
2. Ventilation/perfusion (**V/Q**) scan can be used for screening for a suspected clinical diagnosis of PE.
3. VTE in young patients, family history of VTE and **recurrent** VTE should prompt screening for a hypercoagulable state.

SECOND GENERATION

Bemiparin is a second-generation LMWH with a very low (3,600 Da) molecular weight and long (5.3 hours) half-life. Dose for prophylaxis is 2500 IU SC OD in moder-ate risk and 3500 IU SC OD in high risk cases. Dose for treatment is 115 IU/kg SC OD.

S

SECONDARY PREVENTION

Long-term anticoagulation may be required for the secondary prevention of recurrent VTE in some patients who have had an episode of VTE. This can be done with LMWH or direct oral anticoagulants (**DOAC**s) on an outpatient basis.

SEMULOPARIN

A novel ultra-LMWH that reduced the incidence of VTE vs. placebo in **cancer** patients. Prophylactic dose is 20–40 mg/day.

SENSITIVITY

Sensitivity of a test indicates the false-negative rate (i.e. disease is present but the test is negative) i.e. cases missed, e.g. when the sensitivity rate of Doppler US for calf DVT is 60%, it means that if Doppler US is done on 100 patients with calf DVT, only 60 will be detected– 40 will be missed (false-negative).

SEQUELAE

DVT can result in disabling post-thrombotic syndrome (**PTS**). Sequelae of DVT can be prevented or reduced by the use of graduated compression stockings (**GCS**) for at least 1 year after DVT.

SERENA WILLIAMS

Serena Williams, the famous American tennis player, had an episode of pulmonary embolism (PE) shortly after childbirth. She had had an earlier episode of PE and was on anticoagulants which were, however, stopped for the emergency cesarean section. Later, an inferior vena cava (IVC) **filter** was also placed.

https://www.theguardian.com/sport/2011/jun/13/serena-williams-blood-clot-wimbledon

SGRH (SIR GANGA RAM HOSPITAL)

At the Sir Ganga Ram Hospital (SGRH), New Delhi, India, DVT was suspected in 1,552 patients between 2001 and 2004. Isotope venography proved DVT in 744 patients. Isotope lung perfusion scan showed high probability of PE in 294 patients – 50% of these patients were asymptomatic.

Parakh R, Kapadia SR, Sen I, Agarwal S, Grover T, Yadav A. Pulmonary embolism: A frequent occurrence in Indian patients with symptomatic lower limb venous thrombosis. *Asian J Surg.* 2006;29(2):86–91. doi: 10.1016/S1015-9584(09)60113-5. PMID: 16644508.

SIGN (SCOTTISH INTERCOLLEGIATE GUIDELINES NETWORK)

Prophylaxis of venous thromboembolism, 2002.
https://www.sign.ac.uk/media/1060/sign122.pdf

SIGNS

A red, swollen, oedematous, tender limb is the most common clinical presentation of DVT.

Tachypnoea (70%), tachycardia (30%), diaphoresis (11%), rales (crackles, crepitations) (50%), fourth heart sound (24%) and increased pulmonary component of the second heart sound (23%) were the most common signs in 117 patients with acute PE (Stein. *Chest* 1991). It must, however, be kept in mind that these are all nonspecific signs which can be present in many other conditions and do not necessarily suggest PE.

Stein PD, Henry JW. Clinical characteristics of patients with acute pulmonary embolism stratified according to their presenting syndromes. *Chest.* 1997;112(4):974–79. doi:10.1378/chest.112.4.974

SILENT

1. Both DVT and PE are usually clinically silent i.e. **asymptomatic** and, therefore, difficult to diagnose.
2. PE is a 'silent' killer.

SKIN NECROSIS

Necrosis of the skin can be induced by **warfarin.** It is usually preceded by a skin rash. This happens more frequently in patients with **cancer**. Warfarin should be stopped and vitamin K given; heparin may be used as the alternative anticoagulation.

SMART (SURGICAL MULTINATIONAL ASIAN REGISTRY IN THROMBOSIS) STUDY

The incidence of VTE is thought to be low in **Asian** patients relative to Western patients undergoing surgery. SMART was a prospective observational study performed at 39 centres in 11 countries on 2,420 Asian patients undergoing major orthopaedic surgery e.g. hip fracture surgery (**HFS**), total hip replacement (**THR**) or total knee replacement (**TKR**) without thromboprophylaxis. The rate of symptomatic VTE was 2.3% and of sudden death was 1.2%. The incidence of symptomatic VTE after major orthopaedic surgery in Asian patients was not low; it was consistent with the rates observed in Western countries. The use of thromboprophylaxis should be considered in Asian patients also undergoing such high-risk surgical procedures.

Leizorovicz A, Turpie AG, Cohen AT, et al. Epidemiology of venous thromboembolism in Asian patients undergoing major orthopedic surgery without thromboprophylaxis. The SMART study. *J Thromb Haemost.* 2005;3(1):28–34. doi: 10.1111/j.1538-7836.2004.01094.x

SMOKING

Smoking is associated with a higher risk of VTE. Patients planning elective surgery should be advised to stop smoking for 4–6 weeks before the operation.

SOCIETY OF AMERICAN GASTROINTESTINAL AND ENDOSCOPIC SURGEONS (SAGES)

See **SAGES**.

SOS

SOS i.e. sick, old, (undergone) surgery patients are at high risk for VTE.

SPECIFICITY

Specificity of a test indicates the false-positive (i.e. the test is positive but the disease is not present) rate – these are cases wrongly diagnosed; when the specificity of Doppler US for calf DVT is 95%, it means that when Doppler US shows calf DVT in 100 patients, it is actually present in only 95; in 5 cases, there is no DVT (false-positive).

SPINAL ANAESTHESIA

See **Neuraxial anaesthesia**.

SPINAL CORD INJURY (SCI)

Spinal cord injury (SCI) patients with **paraplegia** or **quadriplegia** are at a very high risk for VTE. All patients with SCI should receive prophylaxis – initially with heparin for 7–10 days and then oral anticoagulation for at least 3 months.

SPINAL HEMATOMA

The use of **neuraxial** anaesthesia along with thromboprophylaxis may rarely (1 in 150,000) cause a spinal **hematoma**. It presents as severe low back pain, numbness and weakness of the lower limbs with bowel or bladder dysfunction. Early decompression by laminectomy may be helpful, or it may result in complete and permanent paraplegia.

SPINAL SURGERY

Not all patients undergoing spinal surgery need prophylaxis – it is indicated in patients with additional risk factors for VTE.

SPIRAL CT

See **CT angiography**.

STANDARD OF CARE

1. VTE prophylaxis has become the standard of care for patients undergoing major orthopaedic surgery e.g. hip **arthroplasty**, knee arthroplasty and hip fracture surgery (**HFS**).

   DVT occurs in 40–60% (proximal DVT in 10–30%) of patients who do not receive prophylaxis.

   These patients should receive LMWH (not UFH) or **fondaparinux** or vitamin K antagonists (**VKAs**). Most surgeons prefer to start anticoagulation prophylaxis 4–8 hours after surgery.
2. While UFH is as good as LMWH, LMWHs are gradually replacing UFH as the standard of care for high-risk patients.

STASIS

Age, **obesity**, **immobility**, **trauma** and **varicose veins** promote venous stasis, which increases the risk of VTE.

STATIC EXERCISES

Postoperative patients are at a higher risk of developing DVT. Static exercises of the quadriceps, calf and toes should be started as soon as possible on the day of surgery.

STEMI (ST-ELEVATION MYOCARDIAL INFARCTION)

Antithrombotic therapy with LMWHs is used along with thrombolytic therapy in the early treatment of ST-elevation myocardial infarction (STEMI). This increases the chances of coronary artery recanalization and reduces the risk of reocclusion.

STENT

DVT may result in narrowing/blockage of the veins. Endovascular stents (Fig. S1) can be placed after **balloon dilatation** in narrowed veins following DVT.

STRATEGIES

The American College of Chest Physicians (**ACCP**) recommends that every hospital should have a formal active strategy in the form of a written document for the prevention of VTE.

There are three strategies for VTE prophylaxis:

1. **Group prophylaxis** e.g. all **cancer** patients receive prophylaxis (disadvantage – some patients who do not need prophylaxis may still receive it)
2. **Default** prophylaxis: Only patients who do not need prophylaxis are excluded (disadvantages – some patients who should not receive prophylaxis may also receive it)
3. Individual **risk assessment**: Logistically difficult and cumbersome (requires additional manpower for risk assessment)

STREPTOKINASE

Streptokinase, a tissue plasminogen activator (**tPA**), is a thrombolytic agent. The dose is 250,000 IU followed by 100,000 U/hour for 24 hours.

STROKE

Patients with acute ischemic stroke are at a very high risk of developing VTE. DVT may occur in the paretic or paralytic limb in as many as 40% of patients with ischemic stroke. PE occurred in 0.8% patients within 2 weeks of stroke. VTE

S

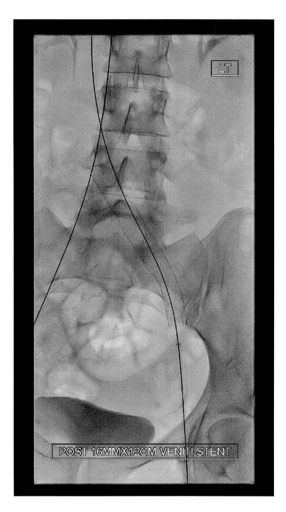

Fig. S1 Endovascular stent in situ in the narrowed iliac vein after its balloon dilatation.

occurred in 20% of patients with acute ischaemic stroke who received **enoxaparin** vs. 35% of those who received UFH.

Hillbom M, Erilä T, Sotaniemi K, Tatlisumak T, Sarna S, Kaste M. Enoxaparin vs heparin for prevention of deep-vein thrombosis in acute ischaemic stroke: A randomized, double-blind study. *Acta Neurol Scand*. 2002;106(2):84–92. doi: 10.1034/j.1600-0404.2002.01215.x

S

In patients with haemorrhagic stroke (where anticoagulation is contraindicated), mechanical thromboprophylaxis should be used.

STRONG

Strong (odds ratio >10) **risk factors** for VTE are **pelvic fracture** or **hip fracture**, **hip replacement** or **knee replacement**, major trauma, spinal cord injury (**SCI**) and major general surgery.

SUBCLAVIAN VEIN

Subclavian vein thrombosis (Fig. S2) is not common. It can occur following the placement of a central venous catheter (**CVC**) in the subclavian vein or as a result of thoracic outlet syndrome because of compression of the vein between the first rib and the clavicle (effort syndrome).

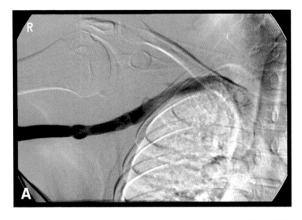

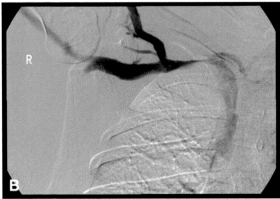

Fig. S2   Subclavian vein thrombosis.

SUBCLINICAL

Subclinical (**asymptomatic, silent**) DVT is common and is the main source of fatal PE, as clinically obvious DVT is usually diagnosed and treated, thus preventing PE.

SUBCUTANEOUS (SC)

All heparins are administered subcutaneously (SC) (NOT intramuscularly). The SC (Fig. S3) injection is made in the anterior abdominal wall at least 5 cm from the navel. A fold of skin is pinched and the needle is inserted at a 90-degree angle into this fold.

SUDDEN DEATH

Many hospitalized patients have a sudden death. Common causes of sudden death are myocardial infarction (MI), arrhythmia and PE due to DVT.

SUPERFICIAL VENOUS THROMBOSIS

Thrombophlebitis can occur in the superficial veins, which are cannulated for intravenous infusions. Thrombophlebitis usually does not lead to PE and does not need treatment with anticoagulation. Superficial venous thrombosis involving the long saphenous vein, however, is an exception; it should be scanned for extension into the femoral veins and may need anticoagulation with LMWH or surgery (i.e. saphenofemoral ligation) to prevent the progression of the thrombus into the deep veins.

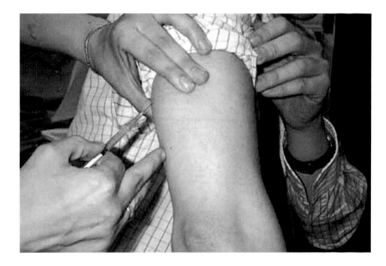

Fig. S3   Heparins (UFH and LMWH) are administered subcutaneously. The injection here is being given in the arm but it is commonly given in the anterior abdominal wall.

S

SUPINE
Supine position for a long time results in venous stasis in the lower limb, increasing the risk of DVT. Bed-ridden patients should be encouraged and helped to change their position in the bed every few hours.

SURGERY
Surgery (especially major, orthopaedic, abdominopelvic, long duration) is a risk factor for VTE.

SURVEILLANCE
Selective intensive surveillance (with **D-dimer**, **Doppler**, etc.) in high-risk patients for early diagnosis of VTE could be one strategy but it is not preferred as it is more expensive than VTE prophylaxis.

SURVIVAL
VTE adversely affects short-term and long-term survival; at 1 year and 5 years, only 85% and 65% patients are alive after an episode of DVT and 48% and 35% after an episode of PE.

SUSPICION
Treatment with anticoagulation can be started even with strong suspicion alone of DVT or PE because documentation or confirmation of the diagnosis may not be possible in all cases of DVT/PE.

SWOLLEN
Current, unilateral and tender swollen leg is suggestive of the presence of DVT.

SYMPTOMATIC
Only 20% of DVTs are symptomatic; the majority of cases are **silent (asymptomatic)**.

SYMPTOMS
Pain (cramp) is the most common and the most predominant symptom of DVT; unilateral swelling of the leg is the next. The presence of symptomatic and proximal (vs. **asymptomatic** or distal) DVT carries a higher risk of PE. Symptoms of PE are tachypnoea, pleuritic chest pain and haemoptysis.

SYSTEMATIC REVIEW
A systematic review is a complete exhaustive summary of the current evidence. A well-conducted systematic review provides the highest level i.e. Level 1 of evidence.

TED

Thromboembolism deterrent (TED[R] Covidien) stockings.
See **GCS** also.

TAMOXIFEN

Tamoxifen, a selective oestrogen receptor modulator, used frequently in patients with breast cancer, increases the risk of deep vein thrombosis (DVT).

TEG (THROMBOELASTOGRAPHY)

Thromboelastography (TEG) is a haemostatic assay that measures the global viscoelastic properties of whole-blood clot formation under low-shear stress. TEG can assess platelet function, clot strength and fibrinolysis, which the routine tests of the **coagulation profile** cannot.

TERATOGENICITY

Warfarin may have some teratogenic effects and is not recommended for use in pregnant women.

TFPI (TISSUE FACTOR PATHWAY INHIBITOR)

Low-molecular-weight heparins (LMWHs) increase the release of tissue factor pathway inhibitors (TFPIs) and thus inhibit the extrinsic pathway of coagulation.

THE-PRINCE (THROMBOEMBOLISM PREVENTION IN CARDIAC OR RESPIRATORY DISEASE WITH ENOXAPARIN)

In a multicentre, controlled, randomized, open study in 451 patients with heart failure or severe respiratory disease managed at 64 medical departments in Germany, venous thromboembolism (VTE) occurred in 8.4% patients with **enoxaparin** (40 mg once daily) vs. 10.4% with unfractionated heparin (UFH) (5,000 IU three times daily) for 10+/-2 days.

Kleber FX, Witt C, Vogel G, et al. Randomized comparison of enoxaparin with unfractionated heparin for the prevention of venous thromboembolism in medical patients with heart failure or severe respiratory disease. *Am Heart J.* 2003;145(4):614–21. doi:10.1067/mhj.2003.189

T

THERAPEUTIC

Treatment of VTE always starts with UFH – bolus intravenous (IV) injection 80 IU/kg followed by continuous IV infusion (18 IU/kg per hour). The dose is monitored with the activated partial thromboplastin time (**aPTT**), which is kept at 1.5–2.0 times normal. Oral anticoagulation with **warfarin** is started after 2–3 days. The dose of warfarin is monitored with the international normalized ratio (**INR**), which is kept at two to three times the normal. Both are administered together for 4–5 days and then UFH is stopped and warfarin continued. Some patients may need to be treated with direct oral anticoagulants (**DOACs**) instead of warfarin.

THR (TOTAL HIP REPLACEMENT)

Patients undergoing total hip replacement (THR) should receive prophylaxis with LMWH or **fondaparinux** or vitamin K antagonists (**VKAs**). LMWH is better than UFH for thromboprophylaxis in patients undergoing THR. Both fatal DVT (25% vs. 12.5%) and proximal DVT (18.5% vs. 7.5%) were less in patients who received **enoxaparin** ($n = 120$) than in those who received UFH ($n = 108$) after THR (Planes. *Thromb Hemost* 1988). VTE prophylaxis should be continued for 4–6 weeks after THR.

Planes A, Vochelle N, Mazas F, et al. Prevention of postoperative venous thrombosis: A randomized trial comparing unfractionated heparin with low molecular weight heparin in patients undergoing total hip replacement. *Thromb Haemost.* 1988;60(3):407–10.

THROMBIN

Thrombin (**factor IIa**) converts **fibrinogen** to **fibrin** and plays an important role in the coagulation cascade.

THROMBECTOMY, SURGICAL

Surgical thrombectomy is indicated if **thrombolysis** is not possible or fails. It is, however, not very useful, as it is usually followed by recurrent thrombosis. It is indicated mainly for **iliofemoral** (NOT infrainguinal) thrombosis with **phlegmasia cerulea dolens** and impending venous gangrene. Increasing pain, progressive oedema, cyanosis and blistering in spite of limb elevation and adequate anticoagulation should raise a suspicion of impending venous gangrene. Thrombus is removed by an **embolectomy** (Fogarty) catheter through a venotomy in the common femoral vein. It can be performed under local anaesthesia also. A completion venogram should demonstrate complete venous clearance. Best results are for an early (<3 days) thrombus; it can also be performed percutaneously with an endovascular mechanical device. A temporary distal arteriovenous fistula may be created between the superficial femoral artery and the great saphenous vein to improve venous patency; the fistula closes spontaneously after a few months. Therapeutic anticoagulation (heparin followed by warfarin) should be given for 6 months. Thrombectomy in itself can, however, cause PE.

See **Embolectomy** also.

THROMBOELASTOGRAPHY
See **TEG**.

THROMBOLYSIS
Thrombolysis can be performed with the recombinant tissue plasminogen activator (**rtPA**) **streptokinase** or **urokinase**. They activate plasminogen to plasmin, which causes fibrin degradation and thus thrombolysis. It can be catheter directed locally or systemic. Thrombolysis is indicated in **massive** pulmonary embolism (PE) with hemodynamic instability or pulmonary hypertension (dilated right ventricle and right ventricle dysfunction on echo). This occurs in less than 10% of patients with PE. The dose of streptokinase for treatment of PE is a loading IV dose of 250,000 IU followed by 100,000 IU per hour for 24 hours.

Thrombolysis of DVT is not recommended as a routine; it is indicated in extensive acute iliofemoral DVT with **phlegmasia alba dolens** or **phlegmasia cerulea dolens** – limb-threatening venous hypertension and imminent venous gangrene indicated by increasing pain, progressive oedema, cyanosis and blistering in spite of adequate anticoagulation. Catheter-directed local thrombolytic therapy is preferred over systemic (IV) thrombolytic therapy. Local thrombolytic therapy results in amelioration of symptoms, prevents pulmonary embolism (PE) and restores venous circulation to reduce the risk of post-thrombotic syndrome (**PTS**).

Thrombolytic therapy is associated with a risk of bleeding. Contraindications for thrombolysis are a current or recent (<6 months) source of bleeding, severe uncontrolled hypertension, recent (within 3 months) eye operation, recent cerebrovascular accident (CVA), ocular or intraocular pathology, intracranial neoplasm, recent (<2 months) intracranial trauma or surgery.

Catheter-directed thrombolysis (**CDT**) using mechano-chemical methods or ultrasound energy (**EKOS**) is now a routine recommendation for the management of iliofemoral thrombosis. These patients may need additional treatment with iliac vein **stenting** for coexisting **May Thurner syndrome**. A similar technique is followed in the case of subclavian vein thrombosis. Various studies have suggested reduction in the rate of post-thrombotic syndrome (**PTS**) without increasing the risk of PE, thus improving the quality of life (**QoL**).

THROMBOPHILIA
Inherited hypercoagulable states e.g. **antithrombin 3** deficiency, protein **C** deficiency, protein **S** deficiency, carry a high risk of VTE; some other conditions e.g. factor V **Leiden** mutation, **prothrombin gene** mutation, hyperfibrinogenaemia, hyperhomocysteinemia carry a relatively lower increased risk of VTE. These patients have VTE at a young age, family history of VTE, thrombosis at unusual sites, **idiopathic** VTE and **recurrent** VTE. Hypercoagulable states produce a persistent thrombophilic situation sometimes requiring lifelong anticoagulation.

Patients with antithrombin deficiency have a 50 times higher risk of VTE and should receive antithrombin along with thromboprophylaxis. Recombinant antithrombin is preferred to that obtained from plasma because of the risk of transmission of viral infections with the latter.

T

THROMBOPROPHYLAXIS

Thromboprophylaxis means prevention of VTE. This can be **mechanical** and **pharmacological**. A large number of randomized controlled trials (**RCTs**), **systematic reviews** and **meta-analyses** have proved that thromboprophylaxis decreases the risk of DVT, PE and fatal PE.

THROMBUS

Clot formed within a blood vessel (vein or artery) by the red blood cells (RBCs), leukocytes, platelets and fibrin. The thrombus can cause partial or complete obstruction of the lumen of the vessel. A venous thrombus is mainly fibrin, while an arterial thrombus contains mainly platelets.

TICLOPIDINE

Ticlopidine is an **antiplatelet** drug that has been found to be useful for preventing strokes and coronary stent occlusions. It is NOT used for VTE prophylaxis.

TIMING

Prophylaxis can be started before or after the operation. If started before the operation, the first dose can be given 2–12 hours before surgery. In moderate-risk patients, low-dose LMWH can be given 2 hours before surgery; in high-risk patients, however, high-dose LMWH should be given 10–12 hours before surgery or started 12–24 hours after surgery to reduce the risk of bleeding. If started after the operation, it can be given 6 hours after surgery; the first dose given postoperatively reduces the risk of spinal hematoma in patients who received neuraxial anaesthesia.

DVT has been shown to occur on day 7 after total knee arthroplasty (**TKA**) and on day 17 after total hip arthroplasty (**THA**) – hence the need for **extended** prophylaxis.

TINZAPARIN

Tinzaparin is one of the LMWHs. It has a higher (6,500 Da) molecular weight as compared to other LMWHs, the half-life is 2.0 hours and the **anti-Xa** to **anti-IIa** activity ratio is 1.9:1. Being a higher-molecular-weight LMWH, it is less dependent on renal clearance and does not need dose modification in patients with renal dysfunction. It has less risk of accumulation and less risk of bleeding in patients with **renal dysfunction**.

Dose for prophylaxis of VTE is 3,500 U SC OD or 50 U/kg SC OD.

Dose for treatment of VTE is 175 U/kg SC OD.

TKR (TOTAL KNEE REPLACEMENT)

In patients undergoing total knee replacement (TKR) without thromboprophylaxis, DVT occurs in 40–80% of cases and PE in 2–7% of cases. Patients undergoing TKR should receive prophylaxis with LMWH or **fondaparinux** or **VKAs**.

The incidence of DVT is greater in patients undergoing TKR than in those undergoing **THR** – it is, however, more frequently distal (calf) and **asymptomatic (silent)**.

TOTAL KNEE REPLACEMENT
See **TKR**.

TOTAL HIP REPLACEMENT
See **THR**.

tPA (TISSUE PLASMINOGEN ACTIVATOR)
A tissue plasminogen activator (tPA) is used for thrombolytic therapy of PE. The Pulmonary Embolism Thrombolysis (PEITHO) trial (Meyer. *NEJM.* 2014) showed that thrombolytics (tPA) improved the outcomes in intermediate-risk PE with a few head bleeds. **Streptokinase** and **urokinase** are two commonly used **tPA**s for **thrombolysis**.

Meyer G, Vicaut E, Danays T, et al. Fibrinolysis for patients with intermediate-risk pulmonary embolism. *N Engl J Med.* 2014;370(15):1402–11. doi:10.1056/NEJMoa1302097

TRAUMA
Patients with multiple or major trauma have a high (about 50%) risk of DVT and PE. PE is the third most common cause of death in patients with trauma who survive beyond 1 day. Trauma patients with at least one risk factor for VTE should receive prophylaxis. The initiation of anticoagulation prophylaxis may be delayed to 24–36 hours after the trauma.

TREATMENT OF DVT
Aims of treatment of DVT include prevention of extension of the thrombus (from distal calf to proximal iliofemoral veins), prevention of embolization of the thrombus, achieve **thrombolysis** to recanalize the thrombosed vein and prevention of recurrence of thrombosis and development of post-thrombotic syndrome (**PTS**). Treatment includes use of anticoagulants e.g. UFH, LMWH, warfarin, factor Xa inhibitors and thrombin inhibitors and thrombolytics.

Short term: UFH 5,000 IU bolus IV followed by 30,000–40,000 IU/day IV (IV infusion 20 U/kg/hour) for 5–7 days. **aPTT** is monitored 4–6 hourly and maintained between 2.5 and 3.5× normal. LMWH (**enoxaparin** 1 mg/kg SC 12 hourly or **dalteparin** 100 IU/kg SC BID) is superior to UFH for the initial treatment of DVT.

Bridge therapy: **Warfarin** (5 mg oral) or **acenocoumarol** (4 mg oral) is started on day 3–5, **PT/INR** is to be monitored. The **overlap** of heparin (UFH or LMWH) and warfarin lasts usually for 2–3 days.

T

Long-term: Warfarin (with monitoring of INR, which should be maintained at 2–3) or LMWH on an outpatient basis for 12 weeks. Warfarin may be replaced with direct oral anticoagulants (**DOAC**s); they are, however, more expensive compared to warfarin and have limitations for use in patients with renal dysfunction.

TREATMENT OF PE

Treatment of PE includes therapeutic anticoagulation (in hemodynamically stable patients with normal right ventricle function on **echo**), **thrombolysis** (systemic and local), catheter fragmentation and surgical **embolectomy**.

TROPONIN

PE is a life-threatening complication of DVT. Elevated levels of cardiac troponins in patients with PE predict a high mortality.

TROUSSEAU (1865) SIGN

Venous thrombosis in patients with **cancer**. Prof Armand Trousseau of Paris himself developed venous thrombosis before he had obvious cancer.

TRUST

ThRombosis ExclUsion STudy (TRUST) is a proposed study to demonstrate the ability of a new **D-dimer** assay combined with a clinical pretest probability (**PTP**) to safely exclude DVT or PE in a 3-month follow-up in consecutive ambulatory outpatients suspected of having VTE.

https://clinicaltrials.gov/ct2/show/NCT03477968

TUBERCULOSIS

Tuberculosis (TB) continues to be common in the underdeveloped and developing Third world and is getting revived in the developed Western world also. Active TB may be associated with a hypercoagulable state and higher risk of VTE.

Antitubercular drugs (isoniazid and rifampicin) **interact** with **warfarin** and potentiate its anticoagulant effect.

TUR (TRANSURETHRAL RESECTION)

The risk of VTE in patients undergoing transurethral resection (TUR) of the prostate is low; moreover, the prostatic bed is prone to bleeding – pharmacological prophylaxis is, therefore, not recommended; early mobilization should be encouraged and mechanical methods should be used.

U

UFH (UNFRACTIONATED HEPARIN)
See **Unfractionated heparin**.

UK (UNITED KINGDOM)
Venous thromboembolism (VTE) is the cause of 10% of all hospital deaths and 3% of surgical deaths in the UK.

UMBRELLA
The inferior vena cava (IVC) **filter** used for the prevention of PE in patients with DVT is also called an umbrella (Fig. U1) because of its shape.

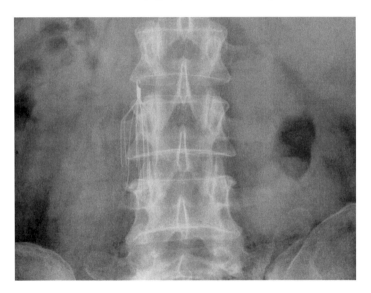

Fig. U1 Umbrella-shaped IVC filter in situ. (Image courtesy Dr Saurabh Galodha, AIIMS, New Delhi.)

UNDERDIAGNOSED
Pulmonary embolism (PE) remains underdiagnosed in many (40–70%) cases because of its nonspecific symptoms and signs and the expensive and invasive investigations required for its diagnosis.

UNDERESTIMATED

U

Incidence rates of VTE are underestimates, as both deep vein thrombosis (DVT) and pulmonary embolism (PE) are very often **silent (asymptomatic)** and are difficult to diagnose.

UNDERUSED

See **Underutilized**.

UNDERUTILIZED

A retrospective review of >150,000 hospital discharges revealed that only a minority of medical patients received adequate thromboprophylaxis (Anderson. *Ann Intern Med.* 1991).

As many as 25–60% of patients undergoing abdominal surgery did not receive thromboprophylaxis (Bratzler. *Arch Intern Med.* 1998).

Anticoagulation prophylaxis, though safe and effective, is underutilized, even in patients at high risk, all over the world, more so in India. Only 50% of 35,329 patients who were at risk of developing VTE in a global 1-point study received prophylaxis – and only 17% in India (Cohen. *Lancet.* 2008).

Prophylaxis was indicated in 466 (95%) of 488 patients admitted to the intensive care unit (ICU) in Jaslok Hospital, Mumbai India, but was used in only 229 (47%) of 466. The main reason for not using VTE prophylaxis in patients in whom it was indicated was fear of bleeding (Ansari. *JIMA.* 2007).

Lack of awareness, nonavailability of guidelines and national healthcare policy and reimbursement issues are other reasons for nonutilization of thromboprophylaxis.

Anderson FA Jr, Wheeler HB, Goldberg RJ, Hosmer DW, Forcier A, Patwardhan NA. Physician practices in the prevention of venous thromboembolism. *Ann Intern Med.* 1991;115(8):591–95. doi: 10.7326/0003-4819-591. PMID: 1892330.

Bratzler DW, Raskob GE, Murray CK, Bumpus LJ, Piatt DS. Underuse of venous thromboembolism prophylaxis for general surgery patients: physician practices in the community hospital setting. *Arch Intern Med.* 1998;158(17):1909–12. doi: 10.1001/archinte.158.17.1909. PMID: 9759687.

Cohen AT, Tapson VF, Bergmann JF, Goldhaber SZ, Kakkar AK, Deslandes B, Huang W, Zayaruzny M, Emery L, Anderson FA Jr; ENDORSE Investigators. Venous thromboembolism risk and prophylaxis in the acute hospital care setting (ENDORSE study): A multinational cross-sectional study. *Lancet.* 2008;371(9610):387–94. doi: 10.1016/S0140-6736(08)60202-0. PMID: 18242412

Ansari K, Dalal K, Patel M. Risk stratification and utilisation of thromboembolism prophylaxis in a medical-surgical ICU: A hospital-based study. *J Indian Med Assoc.* 2007;105(9):536, 538, 540 passim.

UNEXPLAINED DEATH

PE is a common cause of unexplained death in hospitalized patients; myocardial infarction (MI) and arrhythmias are other causes.

UNFRACTIONATED HEPARIN (UFH)

Unfractionated heparin (UFH) – obtained from **porcine** intestinal mucosa – is a heterogeneous mixture of polysaccharides of different molecular weights (5,000–40,000 Da) with a high mean molecular weight of 15,000 Da.

UFH has both **anti-IIa** and **anti-Xa** actions, with an **anti-Xa** to **anti-IIa** activity ratio of 1:1. UFH binds to **antithrombin 3**, an enzyme which inhibits thrombin (factor IIa). It has unpredictable pharmacokinetics and a narrow therapeutic range.

Dose for prophylaxis: 5,000 U q8–12h SC started 2 hours before surgery. Prophylactic use of UFH does not require monitoring with activated partial thromboplastin time (**aPTT**).

Dose for treatment: 80 U/kg intravenous (IV) bolus then IV infusion 18 U/kg 1,000–2,000 U/hour (dose guided by aPTT every 6 hours, with the aPTT target being at least one and a half times greater than control).

UFH has a short half-life, and its action can be reversed with **protamine** – both useful features as compared to LMWH in case a major bleed occurs. Disadvantages of UFH include poor bioavailability, short half-life (requiring 6–8 hourly administration), adverse effects (e.g. bleeding, heparin-induced thrombocytopenia [**HIT**] and **osteoporosis**) and need for monitoring with aPTT. UFH is less effective than LMWH in major **orthopaedic** surgery.

UFH is also used in patients with MI, unstable angina, prosthetic cardiac valves, acute peripheral arterial occlusion and in **extracorporeal** circuits e.g. cardiopulmonary bypass (**CPB**), **haemodialysis**, **hemofiltration**, etc.

UNILATERAL

Bilateral pedal oedema may be nutritional or of cardiac, renal or hepatic origin. Long-standing unilateral oedema may be filarial lymphoedema. Recent-onset unilateral pedal oedema (Fig. U2) is one of the earliest clinical signs of DVT.

UNITED STATES

A reported 600,000 patients are hospitalized for VTE every year in the United States and 200,000 new cases of VTE occur every year – two-thirds of these are DVT (mortality 6%) and one-third are PE (mortality 12%).

VTE causes about 30,000 deaths every year (more than breast cancer, trauma and acquired immunodeficiency syndrome [AIDS] combined) in the United States.

UNPROVOKED

A DVT when no identifiable provoking environmental event for it is evident is called unprovoked DVT; also called **idiopathic** or **de novo** DVT.

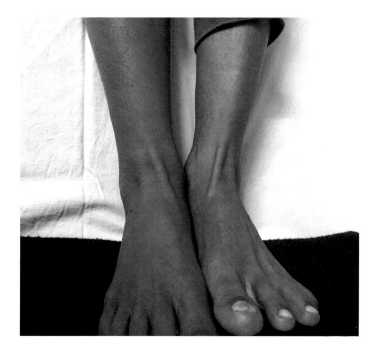

Fig. U2   Unilateral (left) swelling of the calf in a patient with left DVT.

UNRECOGNIZED
VTE often remains unrecognized (and, therefore, **untreated**).

UNSUSPECTED
DVT and PE remain unsuspected in a large number of patients because of the lack of specificity of symptoms and signs; 70% of fatal PE remains unsuspected antemortem.

UNTREATED
VTE often remains untreated (because it is **unrecognized**).

UPPER LIMB DVT
Upper limb DVT is rare and far less common than lower limb DVT; it may occur after IV cannulation of veins in the upper limb or following brachial plexus injuries.

UROKINASE
Urokinase, a tissue plasminogen activator (**tPA**), is used as a thrombolytic agent – 4,400/kg/hour for 12 hours.

UROLOGIC SURGERY

Patients undergoing major open urologic surgery e.g. nephrectomy, radical cystectomy, radical prostatectomy, renal transplant, etc., should receive VTE prophylaxis.

U

US (ULTRASONOGRAPHY)

Real-time B-mode compression ultrasonography (US) is a useful, simple, non-invasive, inexpensive, widely available investigation for **screening** for DVT. Normal veins appear dark, whereas a thrombus is echogenic. Pressure by the US probe will compress a normal vein but not a thrombosed vein.

Sensitivity of US for the diagnosis of DVT (especially in the calf veins), however, is low (about 30–40%). It is more sensitive in detecting DVT in thigh or pelvic veins.

V

VAI
Venous Association of India (VAI) established in 2007.
  https://venous.in/

VAP (VENTILATOR-ASSOCIATED PNEUMONIA) BUNDLE
The ventilator-associated pneumonia (VAP) bundle of the Institute for Healthcare Improvement (IHI) includes venous thromboembolism (VTE) prophylaxis as one of its components.

VARICOSE VEINS
Patients with varicose veins (Fig. V1) have a higher risk of developing deep vein thrombosis (DVT).

VENA CAVAL INTERRUPTION
See **Filter**.

VENOGRAPHY
Contrast venography (Fig. V2) is the gold standard for the diagnosis of DVT. Venography is done by cannulating a vein on the dorsum of the foot and injecting radiological contrast. Venography, being invasive, is no longer used for the diagnosis or **screening** of DVT – **Doppler** ultrasound (US) is preferred; venography, however, is still preferred to document DVT in clinical trials. Nonfilling of the vein, intraluminal filling defect and abrupt cutoff suggest a diagnosis of DVT; collaterals may be seen.

For **radionuclide** ascending venography, 4–6 ci of ^{99m}Tc-labelled albumin macro-aggregates are injected into the dorsal pedal veins of both feet and tourniquets are applied above the ankle, below the knee and in the mid-thigh; imaging is done using a gamma camera. No or poor visualization of a vein, filling defects (if the vein is visualized), collateral veins, visualization of superficial veins plus nonvisualization of deep veins and pooling of contrast are features of DVT.

Venograms can be obtained with computed tomography (CT) and magnetic resonance (MR) imaging also.

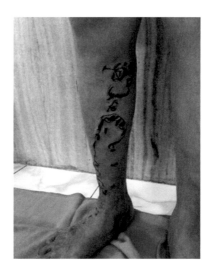

Fig. V1   Varicose veins. (Image courtesy Dr Brijesh Singh, SGPGIMS, Lucknow.)

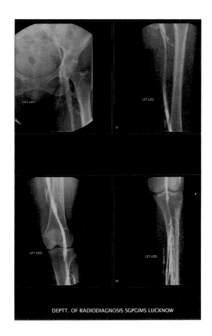

Fig. V2   Venography is the gold standard for the diagnosis of DVT but is invasive.

V

VENOUS COMPRESSION
Venous compression e.g. due to a tumour or hematoma predisposes to DVT. **May Thurner syndrome,** where the left common iliac vein is compressed by the right common iliac artery, may lead to DVT on the left side.

VENOUS ECZEMA
Patients with long-standing DVT can develop venous eczema i.e. hyperpigmentation (Fig. V3), lipodermatosclerosis.

VENOUS FOOT PUMP (VFP)
The venous foot pump (VFP) (Fig. V4) inflates a bag around the foot to a pressure of 130 mm Hg for 3–5 seconds every 20–30 seconds and promotes high-velocity venous flow.

VENOUS GANGRENE
Venous gangrene can occur as a result of **phlegmasia cerulea dolens** and needs urgent **thrombolysis** or surgical **thrombectomy** – left untreated, it may even require amputation.

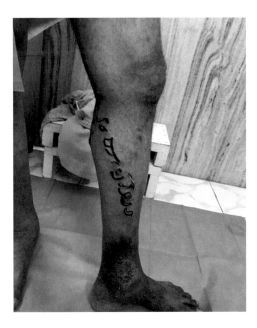

Fig. V3   Pigmentation around the medial side of the ankle (a healed ulcer and varicose veins are also seen). (Image courtesy Dr Brijesh Singh, SGPGIMS, Lucknow.)

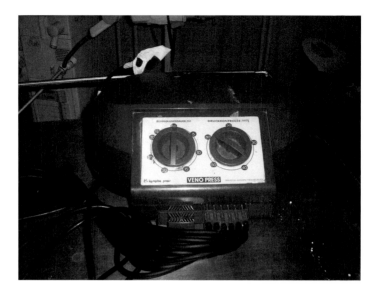

Fig. V4   Venous foot pump.

VENOUS HYPERTENSION

Venous hypertension develops in patients with post-thrombotic syndrome (**PTS**), a sequel of DVT.

VENOUS ULCER

1. Patients with post-thrombotic syndrome (**PTS**), a sequel of DVT, may develop a venous ulcer (Fig. V5).
2. Almost 25% of venous ulcers are caused by the **sequelae** of DVT.

VENTILATION LUNG SCAN

A ventilation lung scan is performed after nebulization with ^{99m}Tc-labelled aerosol.

VENTILATION/PERFUSION LUNG SCAN (V/Q SCAN)

A ventilation/perfusion (V/Q) lung scan is the primary **screening** test for suspected pulmonary embolism (PE), as it is noninvasive. It has a high predictive value – a normal V/Q scan rules out PE (except a large saddle thrombus at the bifurcation of the pulmonary artery). The V/Q scan can be classified as high, intermediate and low probability. A high-probability V/Q scan should be treated as PE, as it has a 90% probability of PE. A nondiagnostic (intermediate or low

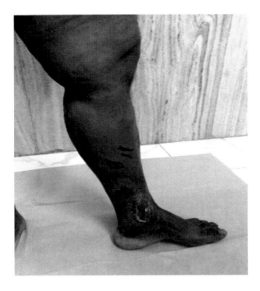

Fig. V5   Ulcer on the medial side of the ankle (pigmentation and varicose veins are also seen). (Image courtesy Dr Brijesh Singh, SGPGIMS, Lucknow.)

probability) V/Q scan, however, needs further evaluation with **Doppler**, **echo** and pulmonary angiography.

In the PIOPED study (*JAMA* 1990), 931 patients underwent scintigraphy and 755 of these underwent pulmonary angiography; 251 (33%) of 755 demonstrated PE. Almost all patients with PE had abnormal isotope scans, but so did most without PE (sensitivity, 98%; specificity, 10%). Of 116 patients with high-probability scans, 102 (88%) had PE, but only a minority with PE had high-probability scans (sensitivity, 41%; specificity, 97%). Of 322 with intermediate-probability scans, 105 (33%) had PE. PE occurred among only 12% of patients with low-probability scans. Clinical assessment combined with the V/Q scan established the diagnosis or exclusion of PE only for a minority of patients.

PIOPED Investigators. Value of the ventilation/perfusion scan in acute pulmonary embolism. Results of the prospective investigation of pulmonary embolism diagnosis (PIOPED). *JAMA*. 1990;263(20):2753–59. doi: 10.1001/jama.1990.03440200057023

VIRCHOW
Rudolf Carl Virchow's (1821–1902) triad for thrombosis includes:

1. Change in the blood flow: Reduced/stagnant blood flow – venous stasis e.g. during immobilization, postoperative period, congestive heart failure (**CHF**), **pregnancy** and **postpartum**
2. Change in the blood constituents: Hypercoagulability e.g. in **cancer**, sepsis, patients on oral contraceptive pills (**OCP**s) or hormone replacement therapy (**HRT**), **thrombophilia**
3. Change or damage in the vessel wall: Intimal or endothelial injury e.g. **varicose veins**, sepsis

VISCERAL VENOUS THROMBOSIS

Thrombosis of the visceral veins e.g. **superior mesenteric** (Fig. V6), splenic, **portal vein** can be secondary to a local inflammatory cause e.g. acute pancreatitis, chronic pancreatitis, in which case it is usually transient and resolves on its own. It may be caused by an adjacent cancer e.g. pancreas, cholangiocarcinoma. If no local cause is present, the patient should be investigated for **thrombophilia** and usually needs lifelong anticoagulation.

VITAMIN K

Vitamin K, along with fresh frozen plasma (**FFP**), is useful to control bleeding in patients on **warfarin.**

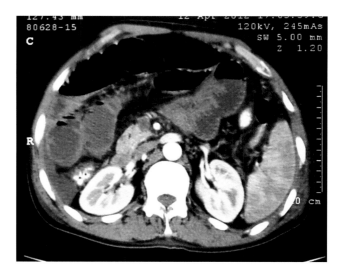

Fig. V6   Contrast-enhanced CT shows thrombus in the superior mesenteric vein.

VKA (VITAMIN K ANTAGONIST)

Warfarin (coumadin) is a vitamin K antagonist (VKA). Other VKAs are **aceno-coumarol** and **phenindione**. VKAs have several **interactions** with **food** and **drugs**. They have a narrow therapeutic window; their use, therefore, requires **monitoring** of **INR** and frequent dose adjustment.

V/Q SCAN

See **Ventilation/perfusion scan**.

VSI

The Vascular Society of India (VSI), established in 1994, publishes the *Indian Journal of Vascular and Endovascular Surgery.*

   https://vascularsocietyofindia.com/

VTE (VENOUS THROMBOEMBOLISM)

VTE includes DVT and PE. About two-thirds of patients with symptomatic VTE have DVT and one-third have PE.

W

WARFARIN

Warfarin, a synthetic derivative of dicoumarol (**coumarin** derivative), is an oral anticoagulant. It is a vitamin K antagonist (**VKA**) and inhibits the synthesis of **vitamin K**–dependent factors i.e. II, VII, IX and X. Warfarin is the mainstay of long-term management of venous thromboembolism (VTE), but it has a delayed onset of action i.e. it becomes effective in about 48–72 hours. For the management of VTE, heparin (unfractionated heparin [UFH] or low-molecular-weight heparin [LMWH]) is started first; oral anticoagulation with warfarin should be started within 24 hours. Heparin is discontinued when the international normalization ratio (**INR**) is >3 for 2 consecutive days. Warfarin is thus overlapped with **heparin** for the first few (3–5) days. Since warfarin has a prolonged duration of action, the therapeutic effect of warfarin may last for a few days even after its withdrawal.

Warfarin is widely used in patients with atrial fibrillation, valvular heart disease and those with prosthetic heart valves.

Warfarin may cause skin necrosis preceded by a painful rash (especially in patients with **cancer**). Warfarin interacts with several **drugs** and **food** components.

The prophylactic dose of warfarin is 1–2 mg/day e.g. in a patient with cancer on **chemotherapy**. This low dose does not require monitoring. Low-dose (1 mg) warfarin reduces the incidence of central venous catheter (**CVC**)–related deep vein thrombosis (DVT) from 38% to 10%.

The therapeutic dose of warfarin is titrated with the INR, which is kept between 2 and 3 to begin with and between 1.5 and 2.0 after 3 months. INR monitoring is done on a weekly basis to begin with – later it can be done every 4–6 weeks. Warfarin has a long (48 hours) half-life; the therapeutic dose of warfarin should therefore be stopped for at least 4 days before any major invasive procedure so that the INR becomes <1.5. LMWH or UFH is started and continued up to 6 hours before the procedure – they are restarted 12 hours after surgery and continued for 3 days. Simultaneously, warfarin is also started, and after an **overlap** of 3–5 days, LMWH or UFH is discontinued when INR is >2.0.

Bleeding (Fig. W1) in a patient on warfarin can be controlled with fresh frozen plasma (**FFP**), vitamin K and/or prothrombinase concentrate, which can also be used if an emergency intervention is required in a patient on warfarin (this is one of the advantages of warfarin over direct oral anticoagulants [**DOACs**]; the other is its lower cost).

Low-dose warfarin with a target INR of 1.5–2.0 reduced the risk of recurrent VTE.

Kearon C, Ginsberg JS, Kovacs MJ, Anderson DR, Wells P, Julian JA, MacKinnon B, Weitz JI, Crowther MA, Dolan S, Turpie AG, Geerts W, Solymoss S, van Nguyen P, Demers C, Kahn SR, Kassis J, Rodger M, Hambleton J,

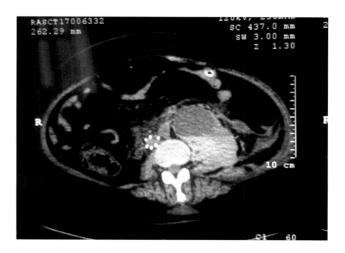

Fig. W1   A large hematoma (hyperdense) with liquefaction (hypodense) seen in the left psoas muscle in a patient on long-term oral anticoagulation with warfarin for recurrent VTE; IVC filter placed earlier is also seen in situ.

Gent M; Extended Low-Intensity Anticoagulation for Thrombo-Embolism Investigators. Comparison of low-intensity warfarin therapy with conventional-intensity warfarin therapy for long-term prevention of recurrent venous thromboembolism. *N Engl J Med*. 2003;349(7):631–39. doi: 10.1056/NEJMoa035422. PMID: 12917299.

Anecdotes

Warfarin is named after the Wisconsin Alumni Research Foundation (WARF), which funded its original research in the 1930s. It was first approved as a rodenticide in 1938.

U.S. President Dwight D. Eisenhower was given warfarin after he suffered a myocardial infarction (MI) in 1955.

WARNING

Massive, and even fatal, pulmonary embolism (PE) usually occurs without any prior warning.

WELLS SCORE (FOR DVT)

The Wells Score is used for pretest probability (**PTP**) assessment of DVT i.e. to predict the degree of risk for VTE and to decide which patients with suspected clinical diagnosis of VTE should be investigated. It must, however, be remembered that it is NOT a diagnostic score.

Active **cancer** (within 6 months), **paralysis** or paresis, immobilization, bed rest >3 days, major surgery (within 12 weeks), swollen entire leg, calf (10 cm below the tibial tuberosity) **circumference** >3 cm than the other leg, collateral (nonvaricose) superficial veins, localized tenderness along the deep veins, unilateral pitting oedema in a symptomatic leg and previous documented DVT – each is given 1 point

The risk is then stratified as follows:

Low (score 0)	Probability of DVT <5% (unlikely) – **D-dimer** is done to rule out DVT; if D-dimer is negative, there is no DVT; if D-dimer is positive, ultrasound (US) should be done
Medium (score 1–2)	Probability of DVT 15–20% (likely) – Doppler US may be performed; if the US is normal, it should be repeated after 1 week
High (score ≥3)	Probability of DVT 30–50% – invasive tests should be performed to confirm DVT

WELLS SCORE (FOR PE)

Points are given as: PE is the #1 clinical diagnosis, 3.0; symptoms and signs of DVT, 3.0; heart rate >100/minute, 1.5; immobilization >3 days, 1.5; surgery within 4 weeks, 1.5; previous objectively diagnosed PE or DVT, 1.5; haemoptysis, 1.0 **cancer** within 6 months, 1.0.

Two models are used:

1. Three-tier model: Score
   - <2.0: low risk, probability of PE <1% – **D-dimer**
   - 2.0–6.0: moderate risk, probability of PE about 15% – **D-dimer**
   - >6.0: high risk, probability of PE about 40% – diagnostic imaging i.e. CT pulmonary angiography **(CTPA)** is recommended
2. Two-tier model: Score
   - <4.0: PE unlikely – **D-dimer** to rule out PE
   - >4.0: PE likely – diagnostic imaging i.e. CTPA is recommended

WINDOW

Ten percent of patients who die of PE die within 1 hour of the onset of the symptoms, thus giving a very narrow window of opportunity for its diagnosis and management.

W

WORLD THROMBOSIS DAY

The thirteenth of October, the birthday of Rudolf **Virchow**, is celebrated as World Thrombosis Day.

https://www.worldthrombosisday.org/about/wtd/

WOUND HEMATOMA

A wound hematoma is a common but innocuous adverse event in surgical patients receiving thromboprophylaxis.

X

Xa, INHIBITOR
Several selective inhibitors of factor Xa are now available; they include **Fondaparinux, Idraparinux** (synthetic **pentasaccharide** that binds to **antithrombin**) and **Rivaroxaban.**

XIMELAGATRAN
Ximelagatran (the prodrug of melagatran) was introduced as a new synthetic oral direct thrombin inhibitor (**DTI**) anticoagulant. It has, however, been discontinued, as it has significant hepatotoxicity.

SUGGESTED READINGS

References

Das SK. New oral anticoagulants. *J India Coll Cardiol.* 2016;6(Suppl1):128–31.

Das SK. Which oral anticoagulant to use: Factor Xa inhibitor or thrombin inhibitor? *Natl Med J India.* 2013;26(4):221–22. PMID: 24758448. http://archive. nmji.in/archives/Volume-26/Issue-4/SS-III.pdf.

Kapoor VK. Venous thromboembolism in India. *Natl Med J India.* 2010;23(4): 193–95. PMID: 21192509. http://archive.nmji.in/archives/Volume-23/Issue-4/ PDF-volume-23-issue-4/Editorial.pdf.

Parakh R, Kakkar VV, Kakkar AK. *J Assoc Physic India* 2007;55: 49–70. PMID: 17444345.

Sarvananthan T, Das SK. Thrombosis simplified. *Phlebology* 2012;27(Suppl 2): 12–22. https://journals.sagepub.com/doi/pdf/10.1258/phleb.2012.012s33.

Snow V, Qaseem A, Barry P, Hornbake ER, Rodnick JE, Tobolic T, Ireland B, Segal JB, Bass EB, Weiss KB, Green L, Owens DK; American College of Physicians; American Academy of Family Physicians Panel on Deep Venous Thrombosis/Pulmonary Embolism. Management of venous thromboembolism: a clinical practice guideline from the American College of Physicians and the American Academy of Family Physicians. *Ann Intern Med.* 2007 Feb 6;146(3):204–10. doi: 10.7326/0003-4819-146-3-200702060-00149. Epub 2007 Jan 29. PMID: 17261857.

Recent (2020) Free Full Text Reviews Available on PubMed

Abboud J, Abdel Rahman A, Kahale L, Dempster M, Adair P. Prevention of health care associated venous thromboembolism through implementing VTE prevention clinical practice guidelines in hospitalized medical patients: a systematic review and meta-analysis. *Implement Sci.* 2020;15(1):49. doi: 10.1186/s13012-020-01008-9. PMID: 32580777; PMCID: PMC7315522.

Badireddy M, Mudipalli VR. *Deep Venous Thrombosis (DVT) Prophylaxis.* 2020. In: StatPearls [Internet]. Treasure Island (FL): Stat Pearls Publishing; 2020 Jan–. PMID: 30521286.

Citro R, Prota C, Resciniti E, Radano I, Posteraro A, Fava A, Monte IP. Thrombotic risk in cancer patients: Diagnosis and management of venous thromboembolism. *J Cardiovasc Echogr.* 2020;30(Suppl 1):S38–44. doi: 10.4103/jcecho.jcecho_63_19. Epub 2020 Apr 10. PMID: 32566465; PMCID: PMC7293865.

Labianca A, Bosetti T, Indini A, Negrini G, Labianca RF. Risk prediction and new prophylaxis strategies for thromboembolism in cancer. *Cancers (Basel).* 2020;12(8):2070. doi: 10.3390/cancers12082070. PMID: 32726933; PMCID: PMC7466093.

Langer F, Kluge S, Klamroth R, Oldenburg J. Coagulopathy in COVID-19 and its implication for safe and efficacious thromboprophylaxis. *Hamostaseologie.* 2020;40(3):264–69. doi: 10.1055/a-1178-3551. Epub 2020 Jun 4. PMID: 32498097; PMCID: PMC7416221.

Nicholson M, Chan N, Bhagirath V, Ginsberg J. Prevention of venous thromboembolism in 2020 and beyond. *J Clin Med.* 2020;9(8):2467. doi: 10.3390/jcm9082467. PMID: 32752154; PMCID: PMC7465935.

Umerah CO, Momodu II. *Anticoagulation.* 2020. In: StatPearls [Internet]. Treasure Island (FL): StatPearls Publishing; 2020 Jan–. PMID: 32809486.

Venous Thromboembolic Diseases: Diagnosis, Management and Thrombophilia Testing. London: National Institute for Health and Care Excellence (UK); 2020. PMID: 32374563.

Vyas V, Goyal A. *Acute Pulmonary Embolism.* 2020. In: StatPearls [Internet]. Treasure Island (FL): StatPearls Publishing; 2020 Jan–. PMID: 32809386.

Waheed SM, Kudaravalli P, Hotwagner DT. *Deep Vein Thrombosis (DVT).* 2020. In: StatPearls [Internet]. Treasure Island (FL): StatPearls Publishing; 2020 Jan–. PMID: 29939530.

BRANDS OF THROMBOPROPHYLAXIS AGENTS AVAILABLE IN INDIA

UNFRACTIONATED HEPARIN (UFH)

Heparin	Brand name	Company				1,000 U and 5,000 U per mL
	Beparine	Biological E				
	Declot	Zydus				
	Hep	Gland Pharma				
	Heparen	Claris				
	Inhep	Sun Pharma				

LOW-MOLECULAR-WEIGHT HEPARINS (LMWHs)

	Brand name	Company	
Bemiparin	Hibor	Elder	2,500, 3,500, 5,000 IU (0.2 mL), 7,500 IU (0.3 mL)
Dalteparin	Daltehep	Gland	2,500, 5,000 IU (0.25 and 0.5 mL)
	Daltepin	Intas	
	Fragmin	Pfizer	
Enoxaparin	BioEnox	Bharat Biotech	40, 60 mg
	Clexane	Sanofi Aventis	20, 40, 60, 80 mg
	Cutenox	Gland	
	Enclex	Cipla	
	Enoxacare	IPCA	

	LMWX	Nicholas Piramal	20, 40, 60, 80 mg
	Qualinox	Lupin	
	Xparin	Astra Zeneca	
Nadroparin	Fraxiparine	GSK	2,850 U
Parnaparin	Fluxum	USV	3,200, 6,400 IU
Tinzaparin	Innohep	Ranbaxy	

SELECTIVE FACTOR Xa INHIBITORS

	Brand name	Company	2.5 mg
Fondaparinux	Arixtra	GSK	
	Fondaflo	Lupin	
	Fondalin	Glenmark	
	Fondared	Dr Reddy	

COUMARIN DERIVATIVES

	Brand name	Company	
Warfarin	Warf	Cipla	1, 2, 3, 5 mg tablets
	Uniwarfin	Unichem	5 mg tablet
Acenocoumarol	Acitrom	Abbott	1, 2, 3, 4 mg tablets
	Sintrom	Novartis	

NEWER ORAL ANTICOAGULANTS

	Brand name	Company	110 mg capsule
Dabigatran	Afogatran	Torrent	
	Dabiclot	Alkem	
	Dabigo	Sun	
	Dabigza	Glenmark	

	Dabipla	Cipla	
	Dabirex	Dr Reddy	
	Dabistar	Lupin	
	Dablexa	Abbott	
	Dabxiga	Lupin	
	Goodflo	Lupin	
	Pradaxa	Boehringer	
Rivaroxaban	Ixarola	Zydus	15 mg, 20 mg tablets
	Xarelto	Bayer	

MECHANICAL DEVICES

Brand name	Company
A-V Impulse Foot Compresion System	Cardinal Health
Kendall sequential compression device (SCD)	Covidien
TED antiembolism stockings	Covidien

INDEX

Italicized and **bold** pages refer to figures and tables respectively.